Serving humanity is a privilege
and trauma surgery is a privilege.

To the people who made me who I am today:
my parents and my wife, Emily.
To my children, who were gifts
from my wife.

To the military men and women
who serve our greatest nation.

TRAUMA RED

THE MAKING OF
A SURGEON IN WAR AND
IN AMERICA'S CITIES

DR. PETER RHEE

WITH GORDON DILLOW

SCRIBNER

New York London Toronto Sydney New Delhi

SCRIBNER
A Division of Simon & Schuster, Inc.
1230 Avenue of the Americas
New York, NY 10020

First Scribner hardcover edition June 2014

SCRIBNER and design are registered trademarks of The Gale Group, Inc.,
used under license by Simon & Schuster, Inc., the publisher of this work.

For information about special discounts for bulk purchases,
please contact Simon & Schuster Special Sales at 1-866-506-1949
or business@simonandschuster.com.

The Simon & Schuster Speakers Bureau can bring authors to your live event.
For more information or to book an event contact the Simon & Schuster Speakers Bureau
at 1-866-248-3049 or visit our website at www.simonspeakers.com.

Jacket design by Ben Wiseman
Jacket photograph courtesy of the author

Manufactured in the United States of America

1   3   5   7   9   10   8   6   4   2

Library of Congress Control Number: 2013042441

ISBN 978-1-4767-2729-5
ISBN 978-1-4767-2731-8 (ebook)

CONTENTS

TRAUMA RED

CHAPTER 1

TRAUMA RED

The sound of the gunfire had barely faded away when I got the text message on my phone: "Heads up. Trauma red. We've got ten GSWs coming in."

My first thought was, Oh, no, not now. Not today.

It was Saturday, January 8, 2011, my first scheduled full day off in weeks. I had just finished a thirty-six-hour shift the night before at Tucson's University Medical Center, where I was chief of Trauma, Critical Care, Emergency Surgery, and Burns— thirty-six straight hours of handling whatever sick, bruised, battered, bloodied, and near-dead humans the EMTs wheeled through the doors. I'd had a couple of shootings, two stabbings, several traffic accidents, a pedestrian run over by a car, a guy who fell off his roof while trying to fix his air conditioner. We do medical emergency surgeries, too, for people who just can't wait, or who have waited too long, so I had done an emergency appendectomy and also cut out a cancerous tumor that had perforated the bowels of a guy who bragged to me that he hadn't been to a doctor in thirty years. In other words, it had been the typical day.

Trauma is a 24/7 business. I had been on call from seven A.M. Thursday until seven A.M. Friday, meaning I'd had to handle all the patients who came through the door, and after that I'd had to work another regular twelve-hour shift, so I hadn't gotten home until Friday night. Having a Saturday off was a rare event, and I was ready for some home time with my wife and kids. But first I needed a little me time—and that meant going for a run around the block. In my part of Tucson, in the mesquite-and-cactus-covered rolling hills north of the city, a block is about six miles around.

And now, shortly after ten A.M., and just five minutes into my run, this: "Trauma red, ten GSWs."

There was a lot of information in that brief message. Under the University Medical Center trauma activation criteria, a trauma code red indicated a patient or patients coming in with any of a variety of serious injuries: penetrating injuries to the head, neck, or torso; traumatic brain injury; amputation of an extremity; traumatic cardiac arrest; and so on. Trauma codes White and Green indicate progressively less severe types of injuries. The codes set in motion a series of steps at the UMC Trauma Center to ensure that the proper levels of staffing and resources are available to deal with them.

"Ten GSWs" was even more specific. "GSW" is short for "gunshot wound." It meant that somewhere out there were ten people who had been shot, ten people who were in desperate need of someone who knew all too well what damage bullets could inflict on a human body, and, more important, someone who knew how to fix it. In other words, ten people in desperate need of a trauma surgeon.

I turned around and started running back home.

I picked up the pace a bit, but I knew I didn't have to sprint. Four years earlier, when I took on the job of creating a Level I trauma center at UMC, I had been determined to put together one of the best trauma teams of doctors and nurses and technicians in the country—and in my opinion, I had done just that. Other trauma surgeons were on duty, and I knew that until I got there they could handle anything that came in.

It wasn't as if we hadn't handled mass-casualty situations before. Even in Tucson, multiple gunshot victims were almost a Saturday-night ritual, and every now and then a chain-reaction pileup on the I-10 would flood the trauma center with a dozen badly injured people. Certainly in my fifteen years as a trauma surgeon, fifteen years in the urban battlefields of Seattle and Washington, DC, and Los Angeles, and as a forward-deployed US Navy surgeon in Afghanistan and Iraq, I had seen more than my share of individual and mass catastrophes. There was no reason to suspect that there would be anything unusual about this one.

Still running, I called my wife, Emily, and had the same conversation we had had so many times before.

"Emily, sorry, but there's been a mass shooting, and I have to get back to the hospital . . . Yeah, I know it's my day off, but I have to go . . . No, you don't have to pick me up, I'll be home in a couple of minutes. Could you do me a favor and put a clean set of scrubs in the car? I'll change on the way . . . Thanks . . . I love you, too."

I knew she was disappointed that I wouldn't be spending the day with her and the kids, but I also knew that she understood. I loved being a trauma surgeon, but for Emily, being married to one wasn't always easy. The job always came first.

I called in to the trauma center to get some more information. Details were still sketchy, but it appeared that a gunman, motive unknown, had opened fire outside a supermarket in a shopping mall, shooting into a crowd. A half dozen people were dead at the scene, and the wounded—maybe ten, maybe as many as twenty—were on their way to UMC by ground and air ambulance. No word yet on the extent or the seriousness of their injuries.

The timing of the thing was actually pretty lucky. Dr. Randy Friese was just coming off his shift, Dr. Narong Kulvatunyou was just starting his, and Dr. Bellal Joseph was making the rounds and caring for the patients in the ICU, so we had three exceptional trauma surgeons on-site. The fact that it was a Saturday morning was also a plus. If the shooting had happened on a Monday morning, the UMC operating rooms might have been crammed with patients undergoing planned surgeries, and since you can't stop a surgery in progress to make room for another patient, no matter how great the emergency, we might have had to make do with the one OR that was always reserved for trauma cases. But since it was a Saturday, we'd have plenty of empty ORs if we needed them—which, as it turned out, we would.

I kept running. My phone rang again. It was Randy—Dr. Friese.

"I'm on the way," I told him. Moments after we hung up, the first patient from the shooting rolled through the doors. It was a nine-year-old girl.

Her name, as I would later find out, was Christina-Taylor Green. A bullet had hit her abdomen, piercing the main artery, the aorta. The first emergency personnel at the scene had performed CPR on her, but she hadn't responded. Unlike with heart-attack victims, CPR doesn't really help people who are bleeding to death; they need to get to a trauma surgeon, and fast. It probably was already too late for this little girl, but the EMTs kept trying, transporting her to our trauma center and performing CPR all the way. Maybe there was a chance.

Dealing with mass-casualty trauma victims is about making choices—often life-or-death choices. The rule is simple. The most seriously injured patients who have a chance at living come first, the less seriously injured come next, and the dead and the certain to be dead have to be left to their fate. If you spend time and limited resources on those who can't be saved, it might cost the life of another patient who could be saved.

It's not an easy choice to make—believe me, I know. In my career I've had to make hundreds of decisions like that. Once in Iraq I had to look into the faces of twelve mortally wounded but still living men and declare them "expectant"—that is, certain to die. They were sent to a separate area and left untreated so I could help dozens of others who could be saved. It's something you train for and practice over and over, but in real life it's not like the drills. You never get over it, and you never forget the faces. But there are times when deciding who lives and who dies is part of your job—and if you think too much about what you're doing, you wouldn't be able to do it.

So, yes, the little girl shot down at the shopping center probably was beyond hope. Under the protocols, a trauma patient who arrives at the trauma center without having responded to CPR for fifteen minutes is considered dead—and this little girl was beyond that time frame. But Dr. Randy Friese hadn't wanted to give up on her. She was the first victim to arrive at the trauma center, and while he knew more victims were on the way, at the moment he had time, the help, and the resources to try to bring her back. This wasn't the battlefield, where helping one apparently hopeless patient might very well cost the next patient his life. Maybe there was a chance she could be brought back to life. She was a little girl. He had to try.

There had been no time for prepping or getting her to the operating room. Moments after she was wheeled into the trauma room, surrounded by a carefully orchestrated swarm of residents and nurses, Randy performed a resuscitative thoracotomy on her, opening her chest and massaging her heart with his hands, trying to get it to start beating again. But it was no use—and now other shooting victims who needed him were starting to come through the doors. Randy had to move on.

Trauma surgery is a hard and sometimes seemingly heartless business. You do what you can, with what you have, in the time you have to do it. If a little girl dies, you grit your teeth and steel your heart and move on to the still living. You cry later.

My feelings about what had happened to this young girl were mixed. Rage that such a thing was allowed to happen in our society. Grief for a life lost so young. Compassion for the anguish her family would go through. I had a daughter myself, not much older than Christina-Taylor, and I knew that the heartache they would have to endure would never go away.

There was one other emotion I felt about this young girl's death, and that was a sense of scientific frustration—frustration that the new techniques we were developing for the treatment of trauma victims hadn't already been available for Christina-Taylor and countless other trauma victims. For fifteen years I and other medical researchers had been looking for a way to stop or at least slow down the dying process in trauma victims, a way to buy them that most precious commodity, time—time for us to repair the damage caused by bullets or knives or blunt force before the victims' lifeblood drained away and their hearts and brains and other organs irretrievably shut down. And we were convinced we had found the answer in the form of "suspended animation," a way to dramatically cool down the trauma victim's body and stop the dying process in its tracks until the damage could be repaired. It's like a pause button on your remote. It pauses you between life and death, giving us the time to sew up the holes you are bleeding from.

I know, it sounds futuristic, maybe even Frankensteinian.

But it works. The FDA would soon approve clinical testing of the suspended-animation procedure on human trauma victims at trauma centers across the country, including mine. Of course, this came far too late to help Christina-Taylor. But I'm convinced that in ten or fifteen years the process will be used in every trauma center, and even possibly by the EMTs in the field, and thousands of lives could be saved—if we devoted sufficient resources to it. Not for the first time, or the last, I found myself wishing that we as a nation would spend even a thousandth as much money and resources developing ways to save lives as we spend on coming up with new ways to take lives.

But I couldn't dwell on that now. Randy called with some more information on the second shooting victim who had been rushed in through the doors, just moments after Christina-Taylor was declared dead. This part was unusual.

"Peter, one of the GSWs is a US congresswoman," Randy said. "Congresswoman Gabrielle Giffords. She's been shot in the head."

Gabrielle "Gabby" Giffords was an attractive, popular, politically moderate Democratic congresswoman who had represented the Tucson area in Congress since 2006. She was married to Navy Captain Mark Kelly, a jet fighter pilot who became an astronaut and a Space Shuttle pilot and commander. The fact that a congresswoman had been gunned down in a parking lot in her home district was certainly a tragedy, and I knew it would generate an enormous amount of news media and public attention.

But the fact that she was a congresswoman didn't make me run any faster—because medically it was irrelevant. Throughout my career as a trauma surgeon, I had always maintained a single overriding principle: everybody gets treated the same. It had never mattered to me—or, as I insisted, to the people who worked for me—whether the patient was a cop or a robber, an American soldier or an enemy insurgent, a rich man or a poor one, a congress-woman or a regular citizen on the street. The courts and the lawyers and the insurance companies could sort it all out later, but in my trauma center, in my operating room, in my intensive care unit, they all got the best medical treatment we could possibly give them.

Randy filled me in on Giffords's condition. She had a gun-shot wound on the left side of her forehead and another wound on the left side in the back of the head. This meant that the bullet might have gone through the left side of the brain. This was bad news and good news.

The bad news, of course, was that she had been shot in the brain at all. Statistically, being shot in the brain means that your chances of dying are 90 percent, and if you do survive, the chances are high that you'll be technically alive but in a vegetative state.

On the other hand, the fact that the bullet might have passed through only one side of her brain was relatively good news to me. It meant she had a chance. If the bullet passes from one side to the other, it's usually fatal, with no chance of survival. The statistics have shown that this results in certain death.

It may sound strange, but the fact that the injuries had been caused by a bullet was also a positive, because traumatic brain injuries from bullets are sometimes easier to handle than other types of brain injuries. The holes caused by bullets can kill you because of the bleeding, but at the same time the bullet hole also allows the pressure on the brain to be relieved. If you have really bad traumatic brain injury from blunt forces instead of penetrating forces, the pressure from bleeding inside the skull can kill you, as the pressure and swelling cause the brain cells to die from circulation being cut off to the individual brain cells. It may even push the brain down and out the large hole at the base of the skull, a process called herniation. Herniation results in certain brain death.

But from what Randy was telling me about the congresswoman's condition, I knew exactly what was going on even before I saw her. It was something I had seen far too many times before.

"She followed my commands," Randy said. "She kicked her left leg and squeezed my hand with her left hand when I asked her to."

"Fantastic!" I said. There was silence. Later I wondered if he was confused by my response. But to me this really was fantastic news. I knew instantly that she was going to live. In just a couple of sentences in a very short conversation, I pictured her entire scenario. She was alive, she had brain function, and the bullet hadn't crossed the midline, meaning it had injured only one side of the brain and it hadn't gone from one side to the other. Most of the patients who are shot in the brain can't function at all and are comatose, and if they aren't comatose they are barely moving or combative.

But the congresswoman could hear and respond, which meant there was a great deal of function still left in her brain. In my mind I could even envision the bullet track. It had injured her left brain, which meant she wasn't able to move the right side of her body. But her right brain was uninjured, which was why she could move the left side of her body. The right side of the brain controls movement on the left side of the body and the left side controls movement on the right side; the brain connections cross in the middle. That's why bullets crossing the middle are so devastating. The speech center is usually in the left side of the brain, in an area called the Broca's area, and that may have been injured or just bruised. She couldn't talk, and that's why she kicked her left leg. She was frustrated that she couldn't talk! She squeezed with her left hand because the right brain was intact. It all made sense.

All this was about as much good news as a person with a bullet through her brain could hope for. It would be days, weeks, even months before we could know what the long-term impact of her injuries would be, whether she would be able to recover her faculties, completely or in part, or whether she would be reduced to a vegetative state. I didn't know what the rest of her life would be like. But I had seen this type of injury many times, and after those first few seconds of talking to Randy I was confident that she could survive.

"Fantastic," I had said—and I meant it.

"Get her tubed and scanned," I said to Randy. "Then line her up while they get ready in the OR for her." In other words, I wanted a tube inserted into her trachea to keep her airway open, and a quick CT scan—a computed tomography X-ray—on her brain for the neurosurgeons. I also wanted to get her lined up in the trauma bay before taking her to the OR—"lined up" meaning the insertion of a small catheter into the radial artery in her wrist, and a large venous catheter into the large vein that courses under the collarbone and goes straight to the heart. That would allow us to give her a lot of blood and other fluids to keep her alive while the neurosurgeons tried to stop the bleeding from her brain. Trauma surgeons in the trauma bays could do the lining up more quickly than the anesthesiologist in the OR, so it would save precious time.

When I got home I ran directly to my car—the clean scrubs were on the passenger seat—and I headed for the trauma center, changing into my scrubs at the red lights I couldn't beat. Some cities issue the trauma center director a car equipped with emergency lights and sirens, but Tucson wasn't one of them. One of the trauma surgeons on my team had gotten three speeding tickets while rushing to the OR when we needed extra pairs of hands for emergency surgeries; the local traffic courts were unforgiving in the matter. But I was in a hurry. I'm not saying I broke any speed laws, but I made it to the hospital pretty darn quick.

As I got closer to the hospital, reports of the mass shooting were just starting to hit the news—and many of the early news reports were wrong, including one that said Congresswoman Giffords was dead. But the full story would soon come out.

The congresswoman had been holding a "Congress on Your Corner" event that morning, a meet-and-greet affair for constituents. She and her staff had set up a table outside the Safeway supermarket in a shopping center in the Casas Adobes neighborhood north of downtown Tucson. Some twenty to thirty people were lined up to speak with her. At 10:10 A.M., a twenty-two-year-old Tucson man named Jared Lee Loughner, armed with a Glock 19, a 9-millimeter semiautomatic pistol, walked up to her and shot her in the head at point-blank range. He then turned the gun on others standing nearby and emptied the pistol's extended thirty-three-round magazine; every round he fired hit someone. He stopped to reload but dropped his spare magazine onto the ground. A woman who was in line grabbed it while others tackled him to the ground. The first paramedics arrived six minutes later.

Five people were dead at the scene, their bodies left in place while investigators from the Pima County sheriff's office—and soon the FBI—took photographs and collected evidence. The dead were Dorothy Morris, a seventy-six-year-old retired secretary; Phyllis Schneck, a seventy-nine-year-old Tucson homemaker; Dorwan Stoddard, a seventy-six-year-old retired construction worker; Gabe Zimmerman, a thirty-year-old member of Giffords's congressional staff; and Judge John Roll, a sixty-three-year-old US District Court chief judge who had stopped by the event to say hello to the congresswoman. Christina-Taylor Green was the sixth fatality.

Thirteen more people had been shot and wounded: an elderly man shot in the left chest and left leg; an elderly woman shot three times in the legs; a man shot in the right ankle; an elderly man who had suffered a grazing wound to the skull; a woman who had three gunshot wounds, including one to the left chest; a woman who was shot three times in the chest, abdomen, and right leg; a woman shot three times in the back and in both arms; a man who was shot in the right arm; a man shot in the knee and the back; a man who had been hit in the face and leg; a man shot in the right ankle; a man grazed in the leg; and a man shot in the chest and right leg. Seven of those wounded, the serious ones, were brought directly to the trauma center, and three were sent to the trauma center after being initially treated at a local hospital. The shooter, who was not injured, was taken off to jail.

Later there would be numerous stories of heroism during the shooting, stories of people protecting their loved ones with their own bodies and dying as a result, stories of people, even some who were wounded, charging the shooter, stories of people desperately trying to help the injured until the EMTs could arrive. Later, too, the justice system would try to figure out the motive for the shooting, to find some reason for it, but it would turn out that there was no reason, or at least no reason that any sane person could understand. The shooter had had a history of bizarre and disruptive behavior, the sort of guy that everyone knew had a mental problem, but in our free society there was nothing anybody could do about it. He had bought a gun at a Sportsman's Warehouse, all very legally, and a month later he turned it on a crowd of innocent people.

It was the same old story. Another nut with a gun in America.

By the time I got to UMC, the pandemonium was building. Ambulances were stacked up a half dozen deep at the trauma center entrance, and air rescue helicopters were landing on the roof. There must have been about a hundred people in the trauma center—doctors, nurses, techs, EMTs, cops. Every one of our seven trauma bays was full, with teams of doctors and nurses huddled around an injured patient. The air was filled with voices, screams, ringing telephones.

To an outsider it probably would have looked like chaos, but it wasn't. Everything was working exactly as it was supposed to, exactly the way we had trained for and done so many times already. My job now was to make sure that it continued that way, to take charge, take command, to make the critical life-and-death decisions that had to be made.

I didn't feel any particular sense of anxiety or stress. I knew that for the victims and for their families this was almost certainly the worst day of their lives, and that for the people of Tucson and the nation this was a horrible and shocking tragedy. But I had spent my entire adult life planning for and handling situations like this. It was my job. It was what I did. It was what I lived for.

So you could say that for me, and for other members of the trauma center team, this was just another day at the office.

Another challenging, exhausting, exhilarating, frustrating, heartbreaking, satisfying, bloody, bloody, bloody day at the office.

CHAPTER 2

A SPEAR IN THE BELLY

When I was six years old I saw my father help a man who had a spear through his belly.

The man was a simple cattle herdsman from outside the village where we lived, a little place in the Moroto District of the East African country of Uganda. Cattle were everything to those people, their only measure of prosperity, and so when someone tried to steal this man's cattle he resisted and the thieves put a five-foot-long wooden spear through him. He was still alive when the local police found him, so they threw him into the back of a battered old ambulance, with the spear still in him, and brought him to the village to see if the doctor—my father—could save his life.

My father was a university-trained physician, a surgeon by specialty, but he treated every kind of malady and mishap that Africa could produce: snakebites, broken bones, accidental amputations, appendicitis, malaria, dengue fever, sleeping sickness; he treated diseases that they didn't even have names for yet. My father was a quiet, soft-spoken, gentle man, and a thoroughly competent one. When a disaster came bumping down the dirt road in the back of a truck or an ambulance, he always knew just what to do. A man with a spear in his belly didn't faze him.

My memory of this is both vague and vivid at the same time. I remember walking down to the ambulance as the ambulance driver and a police officer were yelling in Swahili at someone in the back, telling him to get out. Out came a man with a spear hanging out of his side, front to back. I recognized him because my brothers and I had seen him herding his three cattle up the stream earlier that day. I remember how the man's blood looked almost pink against his jet-black skin as it bubbled up around the wound and ran down his legs, staining his loincloth, the only clothing he wore, a deep red. I remember the yellowish whites of his eyes as they rolled up in their sockets, and how the whole time the man never moaned or cried out or made a single sound. I remember my father gently examining the wound, then helping him back into the ambulance, spear and all, and climbing in with him for the ride to the district hospital a few miles away.

I didn't get to see what happened after they got to the hospital, but my father later told me that he had successfully removed the spear and patched the man up and that he had survived, eventually going back to his village with a bad scar and a story to tell. I don't know if he ever got his cattle back, but because of my father's training and skill, at least he got another chance at living.

Now, I guess at this point I'm supposed to say that from that moment on I knew that I wanted to be a doctor, and more specifically a trauma surgeon. But I didn't. The truth is that for the first twenty years of my life I did everything I could to not be a doctor. The guy with the spear in his belly was just another weird thing that happened in Africa.

My family was not African by birth or culture or race. Instead, both of my parents were born in what is now North Korea, but what was at the time a Japanese colony. The Japanese had taken over Korea in 1910, forcibly occupying the country and doing everything they could to suppress the Korean language and culture, an ancient culture of which Koreans were and are fiercely proud. When my father was born in 1933, his parents, who ran a small sewing and textile shop in a town near Pyongyang, named him Ky Young Rhee, but under Japanese law he officially had to have a Japanese name and be taught Japanese in school. I know my father could read Japanese—I saw him reading a Japanese newspaper once—but I don't know what his Japanese name was, because to his dying day he refused to repeat it. The Koreans may have forgiven, but they never forgot.

The Japanese were finally kicked out of Korea in 1945, at the end of World War II, and without anyone really asking the Koreans about it, the US and the Soviet Union divided the country in two along the 38th parallel. The division was supposed to be temporary, but as the Cold War set in, the northern half of the country came under control of the communist, pro–Soviet Union dictator Kim Il Sung, while the southern half was controlled by the pro-Western regime of Syngman Rhee. (Rhee is a very common Korean family name, and there was no relation between President Rhee and my father's family—although I remember my father telling my brothers and me that our family was descended from kings.)

As small-time capitalists and merchants, my father's parents didn't see much hope for their future in a communist state. They were also worried about my father, then a teenager, being conscripted into the growing North Korean People's Army. Later my father told me how his mother had hidden him in a secret space under the floor of their house when the People's Army came around, and how they had searched the house, pounding on the walls and floor with their rifle butts, but didn't find him—which was lucky for me, because if they had found him I wouldn't be here.

That's always been kind of puzzling to me, how my life trajectory—everybody's life trajectory—has been determined by seemingly small random-chance events: the mortar round that missed, the letter unreceived, the box casually checked on a college application form—or, in this case, the fact that sixty years ago some North Korean soldier didn't notice a hollow sound when he tapped on a floor with his rifle butt. There are thousands of small reasons why a life goes one way and not the other, but I guess you can never unravel it. You just have to chalk it up to destiny.

In any event, my grandparents finally did what hundreds of thousands of other North Koreans did: they packed up my father and his younger sister and headed south. My father later talked about how his mother had sold everything the family owned for a few small diamonds—the local paper money was worthless—which she sewed into the sleeve of his shirt to hide them during the dangerous trip south.

They wound up in Seoul, the capital of South Korea, and opened another small textile shop. But history wouldn't leave them alone. In June 1950, the North Korean People's Army crossed the border and invaded South Korea, forcing the South Korean army and its US advisors to retreat and capturing Seoul in just three days. Although the North Koreans murdered thousands of people during the three months they occupied Seoul—government officials, prosperous merchants and landlords, even doctors and nurses at the National University hospital—my father and his parents somehow survived.

The war raged back and forth over the Korean Peninsula for three years, taking more than a million Korean lives in the process (and thirty-seven thousand American ones). Finally in 1953 the three sides (the Red Chinese were in it by then, too) settled down to throw hard stares and occasional shots across the DMZ (demilitarized zone) that separated North from South, which they're still doing to this day. Meanwhile, the South Korean people tried to rebuild their devastated country and restart their shattered lives.

For my father, that meant enrolling as a student at the National University in Seoul and preparing to become a doctor.

He had always been a bright, smart kid and had excelled at the examinations that ruthlessly determined every Korean student's educational future. The rule was simple: if you did well on the test you moved ahead, and if you didn't, you didn't. End of story. Of course, for my father's parents, having their only son be accepted into the university and then into the medical school was the pinnacle of their aspirations, proof not only of his success but theirs as well. Doctors trained in traditional healing methods, such as herbalism and acupuncture, had always enjoyed high status in Korean culture, and modern, clinically trained doctors even more so. I guess the "my son, the doctor" parental syndrome—and now "my daughter, the doctor"—is pretty much universal.

It was while he was at the university that my father met my mother, See Whan Yang. She too had been born in North Korea, where her father had been a merchant in a small village. Like my father's parents, when the communists took over they also packed up their meager belongings and headed south. I remember sitting there as a kid, wide-eyed, listening as my mother would talk about how at age nine she crossed rivers and streams at night, slipping on the mossy rocks and almost getting swept away, or how she got separated from her parents and miraculously found them at a railway crossing. I was fascinated by the drama and the horror of people fleeing from oppression and risking their lives to find freedom and a better life. Maybe the fact that both of my parents were refugees is why I have empathy for the people today who trudge across dangerous deserts and swim across rivers to try to find a better life in this country. When I think of them, I see my mother and father.

The medical-school track in Korea was shorter than it is here, about six years instead of eight, but it was still an all-consuming grind; nowhere is medical school a breeze. Nevertheless, my father and mother decided to get married, and in the Korean tradition the newlyweds lived in my father's parents' home—which caused some problems. Mothers-in-law everywhere are stereotypically hard to please, but in that category Korean mothers-in-law are in a world of their own. For my mother, a modern-minded, independent person, being under her mother-in-law's thumb was difficult. She also had a growing family to take care of. In 1957 she had my brother, Sang Hoon Rhee, and in 1958 my other brother, Hoon Rhee, and in 1961 she had Meong Hoon Rhee—which is to say, me. (Actually, in Korea the family name comes first and the given name second, so technically I was Rhee Meong Hoon. Meanwhile my middle brother, Hoon, didn't really have a first name, just a middle name, because—well, it gets a little complicated.)

I don't remember too much about being a kid in Korea. I remember my grandparents' shop, where they sold wool that you could knit sweaters from, and all the seemingly infinite bright colors of wool yarn in bins, all a shade different from the others. I remember that the house we lived in was heated in the Korean style with charcoal burning under the floor, and even though it was in the city it didn't have running water. We got drinking water out of a well, and we washed at a bathhouse. I also remember that my father and grandfather were always busy, and my older brothers were in school, and my grandmother always seemed to be cooking, so I was alone with my mother a lot. I guess being the youngest, I was her favorite. I remember wishing that I could go to school, too, like my brothers and all the other kids, but my parents didn't enroll me because they were already planning to move—to someplace that Koreans called "Apeurika," and English speakers call Africa.

Going to Apeurika wasn't exactly the career path that my father had planned. After graduation from medical school, he had fulfilled his military obligation by serving for two years as an officer in the South Korean Navy, and since the Navy didn't have many ships at the time, mostly just small patrol vessels, he spent most of his time working in a hospital in Seoul, sort of a military-civilian internship. (Years later, when I was an officer in the US Navy, my mother was stunned when she first saw me in uniform. South Korean Navy uniforms were exact replicas of American Navy uniforms, and she said it was like seeing my father when he was young again.) After his Navy service my father wanted to set up a private practice, but then as now, that cost money, which neither he nor his parents had enough of.

So my father applied for a government program that sent Korean doctors overseas, and he was accepted. When the government told him, "You're going to Uganda," my father had to look it up to find out where it was. We got on a plane, and off we went.

Uganda had been a British colony until 1962, when it became an independent nation within the British Commonwealth. The population was mostly Africans of various tribes—Baganda, Basoga, Bakiga—but in the late 1960s there were still quite a few Brits left over from colonial days, and English was the country's official language. There was also a sizable population of Indians and Pakistanis, descendants of the thousands of workers the British brought over from India to build the railroads who stayed to become merchants, tailors, restaurant owners, waiters, that sort of thing. In terms of class structure, the Brits and high-level Ugandan government officials were at the top, the Indians were in the middle, and the other 95 percent of the population was desperately poor and at the bottom, scraping out a living with subsistence farming and cattle herding as they had done for centuries. As a doctor's family, I guess we ranked up there somewhere between the Indians and the Brits.

Not that we lived in any grand style. In the first place we lived, in the Moroto District, we lived in a modest, government-issue house. But maybe because I didn't know any better, I remember Uganda as a pretty cool place to be a kid. I mean, there were animals all over the place—cows and chickens and monkeys—and there was junglelike forest to play in, and there were all these barefoot guys in loincloths walking around with spears and machetes. Following the local style, my brothers and I ran around in our underwear all day and made spears and bows and arrows and just generally romped around in the dirt, of which there was plenty.

The only problem—for my parents, if not for my brothers and me—was that there was no school. Every now and then a white guy, a Brit, would come around and try to teach us English, but it wasn't regular enough to do any good. Finally my father begged the Ugandan government to send him someplace with schools, and we moved to a small town called Tororo, on the border with Kenya.

Tororo was an actual town, with stores and a movie theater that showed Bollywood-style movies for the Indian population and British and American movies—mostly westerns—for everyone else. It also had a real hospital, with electric power and running water and a few beds, where my father was the resident surgeon. He learned to drive and bought a used white Opel to drive to work in, the first car my family ever had. In Korea hardly anybody had a car, so for us to have our own car seemed really upper-class. The government house we lived in was on the out-skirts of town and was equipped with running water and electric-ity and "Western-style" toilets. We had a small black-and-white TV that picked up the BBC news and shows like *The Saint*, and we also got a membership in the local country club, where my father played golf and we kids could swim in the pool. We even had a "houseboy"—I guess I should say a houseman—a tall, good-looking African guy named Ugulspa who took care of the house and the garden for a salary of about seven dollars a month.

Still, it was a relatively frugal lifestyle. My mother made all of our clothes to save money, and we didn't have any toys except our homemade spears and bows and arrows. But we had a dog named Puppy and a cat named Kitty, and we had a bicycle that my oldest brother rode with my other brother on the handlebars and me standing on the rear axle.

And finally, at age almost seven, I was in school. My older brothers went to a public school, but my parents enrolled me in a private school that had been founded by English missionaries—strangely enough, Uganda was about 90 percent Christian—and I had classes that were taught in English. The school was one of those one-room kind of places where the kids wore khaki shorts and white shirts and learned their lessons by rote repetition. Dis-cipline was strict. I remember a white teacher with her hair in a bun and horn-rimmed glasses whacking my open palms with a ruler, and since I didn't speak English yet I didn't understand why. I didn't speak any English at all when I started, but within about three months I spoke it fluently.

All in all, then, life in Tororo was pretty good. But then Idi Amin took over as president of Uganda.

Amin was a template for the corrupt, brutal, bloodthirsty

dictators who have caused the good people of Africa such misery over the decades. A former sergeant in the British Colonial Army, in 1971 he took over the Ugandan government in a military coup, promoted himself to "field marshal," and started murdering his political and tribal rivals; hundreds of thousands of people would be slaughtered during his eight-year reign of terror. He also began seizing British-owned property and whipping up resentment among the African Ugandans against the Indian population, calling them "foreigners" and "bloodsuckers." Finally, in 1972 he ordered all of the eighty thousand Indians and Pakistanis to leave the country, even though many of them were third- or even fourth-generation Ugandans. And since we were Asian, we had to leave, too.

And back then, just as it is now, whenever somebody had to leave one country and go to another country, the country they wanted to go to was America.

My father had heard that the US, which in the 1960s and early 1970s was experiencing a doctor shortage, was giving immigration visa preferences to "foreign medical graduates," or FMGs. So he drove to Kampala, the capital, took a series of medical proficiency tests at the American embassy, and passed with high scores. Then he came home and told us we were moving to America. We packed up all of our stuff in a few suitcases, piled into the Opel, and headed for Entebbe Airport. I remember how Ugulspa stood there as we drove away, sadly waving good-bye, and how our dog, Puppy, whom we'd given to a neighbor, ran after us for about a mile, barking and wagging his tail. When you're ten years old, that's the kind of thing that hurts.

A few days later we found ourselves living in a cheap hotel in the middle of New York City.

It was a pretty strange experience for a kid. One day I'm in a little town in Africa, under an endless blue sky, and then all of a sudden I'm in the middle of a huge, bustling, modern metropolis with millions of people—American people—around me. The only thing I knew about America was what I had seen in the movies, and this place sure didn't look like John Wayne country. I really couldn't understand why we were even there; I wanted to be back in Africa with Puppy and Kitty and the chickens and the monkeys.

We stayed in the hotel for several weeks while my father got our immigration papers in order and started looking for a job—five of us packed into a single little room. I'll never forget the name of the hotel—the Hotel Victoria, on Seventh Avenue in Manhattan—because it had one of those vertical neon signs just outside our window that flashed the word VICTORIA every five seconds and filled the room with red neon light. My parents didn't have enough money for us to eat out, so every day my mother would go a nearby department store and buy a cooked rotisserie chicken and bring it back to the hotel room, and that would be our dinner.

Of course, even though my father was a trained and experienced doctor and had passed all of his written tests, the American Medical Association wasn't about to let him or any other FMG just hang up a doctor's shingle. He had to go through an internship and residency all over again. He landed an internship in Passaic, New Jersey, and we lived in a tiny little apartment there for a year, and then we packed up again and moved to Youngstown, Ohio, for his residency in anesthesiology. He had wanted to remain a surgeon, but that would have taken too long, and he had a family to support, so he decided to be an anesthesiologist, which offered a much faster track to certification. It was the kind of sacrifice that was typical of my father: family above everything else. After two years in Youngstown he got a job in Uniontown, Pennsylvania, a town of about seventeen thousand people in the southwestern part of the state, which is the place I've always considered home. As an anesthesiologist he was making good money for the first time in his life, and eventually we bought a new home on the outskirts of town.

From the start my parents insisted that my brothers and I become full-fledged Americans. It helped that I could already speak English, but because I had learned it in a British school at a young age, I spoke it with a very proper and crisp British accent. So to fit in, I had to learn to speak American, which meant that instead of saying "I want a glass of water," I had to learn to say "I wanna glassa wadder." (My father could speak English, too, albeit with a heavy Korean accent, and my mother spoke enough to get around; my brothers spoke fluent English, but because they learned it at an older age they retained traces of a Korean accent all their lives.) My parents also started sending me to church and Sunday school, not because they were religious themselves, but because they followed this syllogism: Americans go to church. You're going to be an American. Therefore, you will go to church.

Of course, it wasn't always easy being an Asian kid in America. (I say Asian instead of Korean because, let's face it, most Americans can't tell the difference between a Korean person and a Chinese or Japanese or Vietnamese person.) For one thing, there weren't very many of us. At the time, less than 1 percent of the American population was Asian—it's about 5 percent now— and the numbers were even lower in Uniontown and the rest of coal-country Pennsylvania. It made us kind of an oddity, something that set us apart no matter how much we went to church or how fluently we could say "I wanna glassa wadder." Because my family spoke Korean in the house, I never took any of my friends home with me because I knew how different we were. It also made it a little tough when I started being interested in girls. It was hard enough finding girls who weren't taller than me—I was pretty short for my age—but I also knew that some parents didn't want their daughters going out with "the Asian kid." I remember when I was in high school there was only one other Asian kid in my class, a Chinese girl whose father was a surgeon, and somehow everybody assumed we would wind up marrying each other—as if both of us being Asians made us a perfect match. It was embarrassing for me—and probably even more so for her.

And sure, we got plenty of the "chink" and "gook" stuff from the other kids. At first I didn't know what "gook" meant, but when I found out it was what Americans GIs called Koreans during the war, I was glad they were at least acknowledging I was Korean. That kind of stuff was hardest on my older brothers, who wouldn't stand for it and always fought back; they were constantly getting suspended for fighting. (Since I was small, I took a different approach. If somebody called me a name I would fire off what I thought was a snappy retort—call them a "dumb hillbilly" or something like that.)

My brothers kept their Korean names, and you can imagine what the other kids did with "Sang Rhee" and "Hoon Rhee." But I got tired of trying to tell people how to pronounce my name—"Meong"—so when I was starting seventh grade at a new school and the teacher asked me my name, I said it was Peter. I had known a kid in Passaic named Peter, and he was kind of a cool guy, so I just picked that to be my name. My older brothers gave me a lot of grief about it, and being older brothers, they started calling me "Peter Peter Pumpkin Eater." Later, when I was sixteen and my family all became US citizens, my father had my name legally changed to Peter Meong Hoon Rhee.

Still, I was never allowed to forget that I was Korean, even when people were trying to be nice about it. In my high school yearbook, everyone would write something like, "To my little yellow friend, Peter," or "to the nicest Korean kid I know." They never let me forget that I was always a little different in their eyes.

But I've never let the fact that some idiots called me a chink forty years ago negatively affect my life, or gotten depressed because some high school girl called me her "little yellow friend." I've never whined about how tough my childhood was, because it wasn't. I lived in a nice house and had a great family and great parents. I was on the high school wrestling and swimming teams, I had a paper route, I was a photographer for the yearbook. I went to the prom—not with the aforementioned Chinese girl— and danced to disco music in bell-bottoms and platform shoes. Despite the stereotype of the Asian brainiac, I did well in school but I wasn't the class valedictorian or anything. (Perhaps in keeping with the stereotype, the Chinese girl *was* the class valedictorian.) Every kid takes some lumps, but overall I had a pretty happy childhood.

In fact, the biggest problem I had in my young life was figuring out what to do with the rest of it.

As you might expect, there was always a lot of pressure on me to become a doctor like my father—although, strangely, none of that pressure came from him. As I've said, he was kind of a laid-back, easygoing guy, and while he insisted that we all go to college, he never tried to force me into any given path. But everybody else, especially my parents' Korean friends, just assumed that I would go to medical school. It seems like from the day I was born I heard it, over and over and over: "You've got to be a doctor. You've got to be a doctor. You've got to be a doctor like your father!" As a typically rebellious teenager, it made me absolutely determined that a doctor would be the last thing I'd become.

But if not a doctor, what? One day my high school math teacher said that since I was pretty good in math, I should be an engineer. I wasn't exactly sure what an engineer did, but it sounded good. Then in my senior year somebody told me that there was this school, Georgia Institute of Technology, that was a good place to study engineering, and the application fee was only three bucks. So I filled out an application, and for my major I picked aerospace engineering, even though I wasn't exactly sure what that was; it was just the first box on the form. I was accepted, and the next thing I knew my parents loaded me and my one suitcase into the car and drove me down to Atlanta.

I wasn't there for even a week before I thought, Uh-oh: this may have been a mistake.

It wasn't that Georgia Tech wasn't a good school; it was. But it seemed like the school professors and administrators wanted to prove that it was just as good as MIT or Cal Tech, and so they worked you like a dog. My first year was almost entirely taken up with calculus—calculus, calculus, calculus, all day and all night long. And the competition among students was fierce. I mean, it was a lot easier to shine in math and science at a high school in little Uniontown, Pennsylvania, than to score top grades at a school packed with math and science geeks from across the country, guys who carried slide rules with them at all times and had already taken calculus. Add to that the fact that there were hardly any girls there—the male-female student-body ratio was about nine to one—and, well, let's just say that it wasn't exactly a party school.

I also started to wonder about the aerospace engineering thing. The more I learned about it, the more I realized that as an aerospace engineer I might wind up spending years designing one bolt for the Space Shuttle or something. That didn't appeal to me very much. For a while I thought about getting an MBA after Tech so I could be the guy who managed the engineers who designed the bolts for the Space Shuttle, but that idea didn't set me afire either.

Meanwhile, the doctor thing kept popping up.

I remember once I was talking to a counselor and he had me sit down at a computer—one of those old things that was about as big as a steamer trunk—and take a career aptitude/suitability test. You had to answer all these questions about what you liked (math? science? writing? history?) and what was important to you (money? social status? family? lifestyle?), and then the computer would spit out what you should be. The first time I did it the computer spit out PILOT and DOCTOR. So I changed my answers around a little bit and tried again, and again it was PILOT and DOCTOR. I must have tried it two dozen times, and every time it was PILOT/DOCTOR, PILOT/DOCTOR, PILOT/DOCTOR.

Well, I wouldn't have minded being a military pilot, a fighter jock, but that was out because I wore glasses. As for the doctor deal, the computer didn't make me change my mind, but it did make me wonder.

Then in my sophomore year we had a resident advisor in our dorm, one of those older students who kind of looks out for the younger ones, whose name was Stephen Dawkins. He was African-American and a really intelligent, squared-away guy, and I liked and admired him a lot. His father was a doctor, a family practitioner, and Stephen was planning to go to medical school after Tech. At the time I didn't even know there was a pre-med track at Tech, but there was, with a Bachelor of Science in Health Systems Engineering. Stephen encouraged me to think about it. So I kept thinking about it, and thinking about it, and then thinking some more, and finally I realized that, yeah, that was what I wanted to do. It wasn't like an epiphany or anything, a blazing light in the sky that spelled out MED SCHOOL! But somehow it just felt right.

So I switched majors, and of course the premed track was an almost unbelievable grind—the first of many. And the competition was even fiercer than in the rest of the school. There were about a hundred guys in the program, most of whom had been valedictorians in high school, total brainiacs. In any given class—say, for example, organic chemistry—the professor would give out just five A's in a class of three hundred students, and it was those A's that determined whether you got into medical school or not. It meant long nights studying and no partying, and it wasn't much fun, but I did pretty well, graduating summa cum laude. In the meantime, I had found a medical school.

When I had started looking around for medical schools to apply to, I heard about a relatively new (established 1970) school in Bethesda, Maryland, called the Uniformed Services University of the Health Sciences (USUHS), which was sort of like a West Point or Annapolis for military doctors. The deal was, they would put you through their medical school for free, and in return you had to serve as a doctor in the active duty military or the US Public Health Services for at least seven years afterward. Not only that, they also made you an officer and actually paid you a junior officer's salary—at the time about $20,000 a year—while you were going through your medical training.

That all sounded pretty good, so I applied to USUHS and was accepted. On one of the forms they asked me what branch of service I wanted to be in—Air Force, Army, Navy (which provides medical personnel for the Marines as well), or the US Public Health Service Commissioned Corps, which provided medical care for the Coast Guard and performed other public health functions. Since my father had been in the Navy, I decided I might as well be in the Navy, too.

So that was that. I was going to be a doctor after all.

I remember when I had first called my father from Tech and told him I had decided to switch to premed and then go to medical school. He didn't say much at the time, just gave me some useful advice on how to go about it. But I know now that the minute he hung up the phone he did a little dance of joy. You see, he had always hoped that I would become a doctor, but he knew that the road to becoming one would be too long and too hard if I thought I was simply fulfilling other people's expectations. To make it through, he knew that I had to be chasing my own dreams and aspirations, not his. I realize now just how smart my father was—and how the older I got, the smarter he became. It's funny how that happens.

My father would give me a lot of good advice in the years ahead, on school, on medicine, on life. (In fact, it was my father who first told me about the program at USUHS.) He lived to see me become a doctor, but sadly, in 1999, just three months after he retired, he developed brain cancer and went through three hard years of chemotherapy and radiation therapy. In the end I made the decision to stop the treatment and take him off the ventilator, and my mother and I stood by his bedside for a week as his life slowly ebbed away. He was just sixty-six when he died.

I miss him to this day. And I understand now, even if I didn't at the time, how much his character and integrity and work ethic had influenced me.

So maybe I was wrong in what I said before. Maybe seeing my father take care of that man with the spear in his belly when I was six years old actually did change my life. Maybe seeing him display the skill and knowledge and coolness of head required to save a life in mortal danger really did unconsciously set me on the path to becoming a trauma surgeon.

Because figuratively speaking, every minute of every day, somebody somewhere is getting a spear in the belly.

And someone has to know how to take it out.

CHAPTER 3

NAVY DOC

Our patrol moved slowly through the eerie, pitch-black woods, weapons at the ready. The squad's orders were simple to understand but incredibly difficult to carry out: proceed behind enemy lines to the specified map coordinates, find the downed and injured pilot, treat his wounds, and bring him back. Oh, and while you're at it, try not to let the enemy kill you.

We knew the enemy was out there, somewhere, but spotting him before he could spot us was going to be tough in these dark woods. (This was before US troops were routinely issued night-vision goggles.) And of course, as it always seems to be in war, the weather was terrible, with rain coming down in sheets, thunder booming and lightning flashing, the wind howling and whipping through the tree branches. We had to slowly feel our way through the thorny brush, each man's hand on the pack of the man in front of him so we wouldn't get separated.

And then, suddenly, illuminated in a quick flash of lightning, there they were—the enemy! They saw us at the same time we saw them, a dozen of us staring at a dozen of them. Five seconds later the night was filled with the hot bright spurts of muzzle flashes and the sharp cracks of M16 fire. BAM BAM BAM BAM BAM BAM BAM! It was a full-on firefight, and we kept shooting, magazine after magazine, until we ran out of ammo.

Then we ran over to the enemy and started arguing like a bunch of little kids.

"You're dead!"

"No, *you're* dead!"

"I got you!"

"I got you first!"

It was an exercise, of course, with blanks for bullets and the "enemy" being another squad of trainees like us. The training cadre had made sure that our paths would cross so we would all take "casualties" that we would have to treat and evacuate. It was all part of the military's efforts to turn a bunch of geeky would-be doctors into medical superwarriors—or at least to make sure that in an emergency we might be able to read a compass and take a walk in the woods without getting ourselves hopelessly lost.

Now, I want to make it clear at this point that I have nothing but admiration and respect for the institution and personnel of the US military in general, and of the Navy in particular. The Navy gave me a lot of opportunities in life, and I was always proud and honored to wear its uniform. So anything I say in this book that's critical about the Navy's policies or training or procedures has to be viewed in that light. And remember, military guys have been bitching and moaning about the high command since a caveman first picked up a club—and as any military commander will tell you, it's when the troops stop bitching and moaning that you have to worry about their morale.

With that said, I have to admit that at first I hated the military lifestyle.

My military career had begun right after the graduation ceremonies at Georgia Tech were over. While everybody else was leaving for postgrad vacations, I had thrown everything I owned into my 1975 Toyota hatchback and driven up to Rhode Island to report for six weeks' training at the Navy's Direct Commission Officer Indoctrination Course at Naval Station Newport. The DCOIC program was where current or future doctors, dentists, pharmacists, lawyers, and other professional types learned the basics of how to be Navy officers. I took the oath, was sworn in as an ensign (the Navy's lowest officer rank), and got a GI haircut. Then they marched us to the uniform shop and made us buy our uniforms. That's right, buy. Officers have to buy their own uniforms, and since there are so many different ones—khakis, dress blues, dress whites—it's pretty expensive, several paychecks' worth. This would be a recurring theme throughout my time in the military: first they pay you, and then you have to pay them back. You're in the Navy now!

The indoctrination program wasn't exactly like the boot camp portrayed in movies like *Full Metal Jacket*; we weren't a bunch of eighteen- and nineteen-year-old kids training to become killers. Sure, there was some basic military stuff: PT (physical training), white-glove barracks inspections, Navy officers yelling at you, that sort of thing. We did a lot of marching. Anywhere we went we had to march: whether as a platoon or even if we walked in pairs to the store, we had to be in step.

But mostly it was kind of a military etiquette school. We had to learn how to salute, and who to salute, and how to wear the uniforms. We had to learn Navy history and traditions, Navy regulations and the rudiments of military law, how to say "oh-eight thirty" or "sixteen hundred" instead of eight thirty A.M. or four P.M.—and, yes, we had to learn the words to "Anchors Aweigh!" The hardest part was learning how to be patient and tolerant, how to conduct yourself as an officer. The Navy's thinking was that even though we were going to work in professional capacities as doctors or lawyers, we had to act like officers. That was extremely important in military medicine.

Meanwhile, the physical part of it really wasn't that tough, and neither was the academic part. All that the guys in my platoon wanted to do was pass, which we did—although my platoon was ranked dead last out of a dozen platoons. Compared with, say, the grind I went through back at Tech preparing for the MCAT (Medical College Admission Test), this was a breeze, just a temporary stop on my way to the real challenge: medical school at the Uniformed Services University of the Health Sciences.

The Uniformed Services University of the Health Sciences School of Medicine is situated in Bethesda, Maryland, on the grounds of what was then called Bethesda Naval Hospital. (The Naval Hospital has since combined with the Army and the other services to become Walter Reed National Military Medical Center.) There were about 150 men and women in our class in the USUHS School of Medicine from the Navy, Army, and Air Force, and a couple from the Public Health Service. About a third of them were "prior service" guys who had already served as enlisted men or officers in the military or had graduated from one of the military academies—West Point, Annapolis, the Air Force Academy—and had decided to go to medical school. The academy guys were the gung ho types, the guys who thrived on the military lifestyle. The rest of us were recent college graduates who just wanted to be doctors and didn't thrive on the military part of it at all.

But they never let us forget that we were active duty military officers. Although we lived in apartments off campus, we had regular formations, and we were in uniform every day, in class and in the lab. In the summertime they would send us down to the Marine Corps base in Quantico, Virginia, for field training—

weapons, combat medical skills, land navigation, and how to operate a radio. Again, some of the guys were really into it and would get mad at the rest of us for making too much noise in the woods or whining about the heat or the cold or the rain or just about everything. I managed to win an Expert Field Medical Badge, which is actually an Army badge, and which wasn't easy to get.

But the truth is I didn't take the military stuff all that seriously. Most of us didn't—but, hey, none of us ever imagined that someday we would actually be in a war.

As for the medical-school academics, initially it was an all-out slog. For the first two years it was all classroom work, in anatomy, physiology, microbiology, parasitology, epidemiology, disease processes, and on and on and on. They would give you a huge mass of material and you would just have to sit down and memorize it. I would study until three A.M. and then have to be in formation at seven A.M. It was pretty miserable, and I didn't really excel at it. But I learned early on that your classroom grades didn't determine the future of your career. There was even an equation for it—"C = MD"—meaning that as long as you passed a class with a C or better you would get your medical degree. Of course, this was medical school, so just getting the C's was hard enough, requiring a tremendous amount of work and brutal hours. Most other medical schools in the country had switched to a pass-fail grading system to minimize competitiveness, but USUHS stuck with the competitive grade system.

But then in the third and fourth years things got better. That's when we actually got to see what being a doctor was really all about—and from that point on, I knew I had made the right choice.

The way it works in medical school is that during your last two years, you go through "rotations" in the various departments of a teaching hospital—operating room, emergency room, intensive care, et cetera. During your rotations you do service in all the major medical specialties—surgery, internal medicine, pediatrics, anesthesiology, obstetrics and gynecology, urology, neurology, radiology, everything. It's a hands-on thing. You do physical exams, take medical histories, move patients around, draw blood, gather lab results, draw up patient charts, sew up incisions, whatever they'll let you do—and all the time you're watching what the doctors and residents and interns are doing. At first the residents or interns you're working under supervise you pretty closely, but once they trust you, once they decide that you aren't going to screw up and kill somebody, they start giving you more and more responsibility.

And I found that I was good at it. When a resident or an intern needed an EKG or a Gram's stain (a test for infection) in a hurry, more and more they would turn to me to get it done. Unlike in the classroom, in your rotations you weren't judged by how much information you had memorized or how well you could regurgitate five tables of bacteria or the fourteen different cancers of the liver. Instead you were judged by what you could do, how well and how fast you accomplished a task, how you got stuff done. They didn't care how hard you tried, they didn't want excuses, they wanted results—and they taught me that patients would expect the same. It was hard work, physically, and the hours were long, but it was exhilarating.

The only real shortcoming I had was in the personal interaction with patients. I was introverted and almost pathologically shy, not really good at small talk, and a lot of people didn't get my deadpan sense of humor. It wasn't easy learning how to approach people and start a conversation and start to learn intimate details of their lives, which is a vitally important part of being a doctor. The university gave us seemingly endless classes on how to interact with patients, and they did a really good job teaching us how to talk to people. I worked at it, and I got better at it, but I never enjoyed the one-on-one interaction necessary to be, say, a family medicine practitioner.

Which brings up another issue. There are times when it may seem as though I view sick or injured people not as living, breathing humans with feelings and emotions and people who love them, but simply as cases, as problems to be solved. And that is absolutely true. It's not that I don't have empathy, but the hard fact is that as a doctor, and especially as a trauma surgeon, too much empathy can get in the way of your job and cause you to make decisions based not on sound medical judgment but on your own emotions. Sure, I've seen things that even years later can still make me choke up when I think of them: a little girl shot and killed, a shattered young Marine who shouldn't have died but did. But you can't choke up in the ER or the operating room. To be effective as a trauma surgeon, you have to put a layer of Kevlar around your heart.

Of course, as I was going through my rotations I was still a long way from being a trauma surgeon. In fact, for a long time I was pretty sure that was what I wasn't going to be.

Part of the reason you go through service in the various medical specialties is to make you a well-rounded doctor with basic knowledge of all fields of medicine. But another reason is to let you figure out what you want to be, to see which specialty appeals to you and what you're good at. And while there certainly are exceptions, there are certain stereotypes about what kind of people go into what specialties.

For example, people who go into anesthesiology or radiology or dermatology are often financially and socially motivated; the pay is good, the hours are regular, you can have a nice, easy family life. Pediatrics and OB-GYN are for the friendly, caring types who truly like people. Psychiatry attracts introspective types—some might say you have to be a little nuts yourself to go into psychiatry—while the studious, detail-oriented types are drawn to internal medicine. Surgery, which is the hardest and most demanding track to take in terms of training, is for the brash, confident guys, the type A's, guys who like to be in control. While other medical specialists are often people who work to live, surgeons live to work.

I wasn't sure which category I fell into. At first I decided to go with anesthesiology, partly because of the money and partly because of my father, who had been a surgeon and went into anesthesia when he came to the United States. But when I went through my anesthesiology service, working with anesthesiologists and observing what they did, I realized that they were pretty much on the sidelines, that the surgeon was the guy in charge. I was paying more attention to what the surgeons were doing, and learning how to keep a patient asleep seemed to interest me less and less. Brain and logic said anesthesiology, but heart and emotions said surgery.

Choosing a specialty is arbitrary in some ways. My first rotation was in obstetrics and gynecology, but they really didn't let me or the other med students do much since we were just starting. If I'd done my OB-GYN rotation later I might have gotten to do more, and maybe I would have been more interested in that field. But as it was I spent a lot of time not delivering babies but delivering take-out pizzas to the residents and interns.

Then when I was doing my urology service, the interns and residents really liked me, so they kept recruiting me, telling me what a great life it was. I had pretty much made my mind up—I'm going to be a urologist!—but then I got ticked off at the head of the urology department, who frankly was a jerk, and then it was so long, urology. If I had rotated on urology at a different time and at another location, maybe it would have been different.

Meanwhile, although I didn't realize it at the time, there were two things that were drawing me toward being a surgeon. One was that I had found I had what surgeons call "good hands," the ability to perform a manual task with absolute certainty and steadiness. It's a spatial thing, a kind of three-dimensional mentality; my eyes send my brain a picture, my brain tells my hands what to do, and then my hands just do it, naturally, seemingly effortlessly. Knowing what to do as a surgeon is a skill that you can learn, but surgery is an art as well as a science; being able to make that cut exactly the way you know it should be done is a natural talent. In my case, it was at least partly a gift from my mother, a very talented artist who has that same brain-to-hands coordination. Some people can be taught the manual skills, but it is fairly clear who has great skills and who doesn't. Manual skills always came easy to me.

The fact that as a surgeon I would be cutting into living human flesh never bothered me. Maybe because of my father, I was never squeamish about wounds or surgical procedures. But a lot of my medical-school colleagues were, at least initially. We had all dissected frogs and studied dissected human organs and things like that, but I guess there's just something about seeing a scalpel cut through a person's skin that gives some people the willies. I would estimate that at least one of every five med students I knew got seriously woozy or even passed completely out the first time they watched a major surgical procedure. But I not only enjoyed watching surgeries, I wanted to actually do them.

Of course, as a medical student I didn't get to perform any major surgeries. But when I was doing my surgery rotation at Portsmouth Naval Hospital, learning what the life of a surgeon was all about, the residents and interns I worked under seemed to take a liking to me, and as they came to trust me they let me perform more and more complicated procedures. I was especially good with closings, the sewing up of incisions. Frankly, I could sew them up better, cleaner, more neatly than the residents did, because they were busy and wanted to quickly move on to the next task. So pretty soon the attending physicians started calling on me to do the closings. "Hey, Peter, take care of this one," or "Hey, Peter, close this one up." Like I said: good hands.

The other thing that was drawing me toward trauma surgery was that I discovered I liked action and excitement, liked the feeling of being able to walk into a tough situation and take control. I found this out between my second and third years of medical school at USUHS, when we were all required to spend the summer on TDY (temporary duty) getting military experience in our respective service branches. For example, the med students who were Air Force might spend time with an F-18 squadron, while the Army guys might go to airborne school to get their jump wings or be assigned to an infantry unit as part of their medical team. Navy guys like me could go to sea on a ship, go train with Navy pilots, or go with the Marines, who as part of the Navy depended on Navy doctors for their medical needs. I decided to go with the Marines.

There was a personal reason for that. My older brother Luke (he had Americanized his name by then) was a Marine. Just before I started medical school, Luke had finally managed to graduate from college and joined the Marines. He went to Officer Candidates School, and then The Basic School, and had been assigned as a platoon commander in an infantry company at Camp Pendleton, California. I managed to get myself assigned to his company during my summer training months.

It turned out to be great fun. I got to shoot every kind of weapon—M16s, machine guns, grenade launchers, mortars—and go on marches and sleep under the stars and eat MREs (Meals

Ready to Eat) and call in air strikes, everything that Marine officers did. It was different from the field exercises at Quantico that I had hated so much, because I wasn't working with a bunch of other green trainees but with real professionals, guys who really knew their stuff—including my brother. Luke was an intense Marine infantry officer, and he made sure that I would not embarrass myself or him. He made sure I was squared away, that my hats were pressed and starched—I used up several cans of starch on my hats alone—that my insignias were displayed exactly to regulation, and that I looked sharp. Everything had to be absolutely perfect.

And in dealing with Luke and those other hard-core Marines, I discovered that I had what it takes to be a leader.

Now, we're accustomed these days to describing the young men and women in our military as "heroes"—and in combat they are. But they're also eighteen- and nineteen- and twenty-year-old kids, which means that just like their civilian counterparts, they tend to do dumb things—and that's especially true of the Marine infantrymen, the "grunts." Unlike a lot of kids in the military, the grunts I was dealing with didn't join the Marines and choose the infantry to learn a civilian trade or even, for the most part, to get money for college. They joined the grunts so they could shoot guns and blow shit up. So while in the field they were tough, well trained, and professional, in the barracks and off base a lot of them were disasters waiting to happen. They would get drunk and get into fights and marry exactly the wrong girls and drive too fast and generally do things that would make a parent—or an officer—tear his hair out. I had no idea that being a platoon officer required so much parenting. My brother seemed to be going to the local police station all the time to bail out one of his guys.

Obviously, you want some of those wild-kid tendencies in an infantryman. A meek, introspective kid with a highly developed appreciation for consequences isn't going to be a tiger in a firefight. But that wildness has to be channeled and controlled; somebody has to take charge and tell those kids what they can and can't do. That's what officers and NCOs are for. They have to make sure that discipline is absolute, that their Marines are dedicated and committed to the Corps. When you tell some Marines to charge a hill, you can't have a debate, you have to know that they will take orders without question.

And during that summer I discovered that I could do that, that I could handle those tough young kids—although when I say "kids" I should note that they were really only three or four years younger than me. Although I wasn't in direct command of a platoon, I was still an officer and had to take charge when necessary.

I remember this one young lance corporal, a kid from Montana, who was a totally squared-away Marine in the field but a total wiseass in the barracks and company area, always mouthing off and testing the limits. I asked my brother why he put up with the guy, why he didn't throw him out of the Marines. His answer was that he was the platoon's "best shooter." The Marine Corps has its priorities.

Anyway, I was walking by him and some of his buddies one day and all of a sudden he started making what I guess he thought were "Chinese" noises—"Ching hung chow chung," a clear reference to my ethnic background. Well, I could have let it pass, acted like I didn't hear it. But when a good officer, a good leader, sees a problem he confronts it—and fixes it. Otherwise it's just going to get worse. So I jacked up this young lance corporal, put him at attention, and gave him a thoroughly comprehensive ass-chewing: "Marine, you'd better get your freaking head out of your freaking ass or you're gonna freaking wish that you had never been freaking born"—except of course I didn't use the word *freaking*. The language may not have been particularly officerly and gentlemanly, but it got the point across. I'm not saying that

that young Marine never made his Chinese noises anymore, but he sure as hell didn't make them within earshot of me. And the word got around to the other Marines: Don't mess with Ensign Rhee. Rhee's a hard bastard.

And that's part of what it takes to be a trauma surgeon, and especially the chief of a trauma unit. You have to be able to take charge, make decisions, bark out orders, demand excellence from your subordinates—and when a life is on the line, you can't always be delicate and sensitive about it.

Anyway, in addition to my time at Camp Pendleton, there was another experience that attracted me to the excitement and adrenaline of trauma surgery—although, again, I didn't realize it at the time. That was in my fourth year at USUHS, when I did my rotation in the emergency room (ER).

Although a lot of the rotations at USUHS were done at military hospitals, the Navy also let us do rotations at civilian teaching hospitals. I had always liked traveling and seeing different places, so whenever I could, I chose to get out of the Washington, DC, area and do a rotation elsewhere. My best friend in medical school was in the Air Force, and he and I signed up for more out-of-town rotations than anyone else. We did the absolute minimum in the DC area. For the ER rotation, my buddy and I decided on Charity Hospital in downtown New Orleans.

Just being in New Orleans was kind of an eye-opener for a small-town kid like me. The dorms that we were assigned to were pretty interesting. My buddy and I slept on tiny mattresses on the floor in a cheap room near the hospital, in a building whose first floor was occupied by a business called Wig World. As you might expect in the Big Easy, Wig World had a pretty eclectic clientele. But the ER at Charity Hospital was an even bigger eye-opener.

Charity was one of the oldest hospitals in the US. Its original building dated back to 1736, but the new building was a 1930s art deco high-rise on Tulane Avenue in downtown New Orleans. As the name implies, its primary function was as a tax-funded public-service hospital for underprivileged people and others without medical insurance. A lot of its patients were homeless people who lived on the streets. It also had one of the busiest, if not the busiest, Level I trauma centers in the country.

A word here about emergency rooms and trauma centers. They aren't the same thing. A regular hospital ER is staffed and equipped to handle minor medical emergencies on its own. If you have a broken finger, a cut, or a bad case of the flu, the ER doctor will treat you right there. If you come in with a major or life-threatening medical condition—heart attack, appendicitis, whatever—the ER doctors and staff will try to stabilize you and then call in a cardiologist or an internist or a surgeon to admit you to the hospital and give you the necessary care. Sometimes they'll transfer you to another hospital that is better equipped to handle your condition.

Meanwhile, a trauma center is a section of a hospital emergency department that has the full range of staff and equipment needed to treat patients with traumatic injuries, no matter how severe. (There are actually four levels of trauma centers, I through IV, but here I'm talking about Level I.) A Level I trauma center is required to have a certain number of surgeons, emergency physicians, and anesthesiologists always on duty, with other specialists— orthopedists, cardiothoracic surgeons, neurosurgeons, and so on—easily available on call twenty-four hours a day. Level I trauma centers also have their own operating rooms that are reserved for trauma patients. Any injury or life-threatening medical condition that comes into a trauma center can be treated right there, without having to send the patient to another medical facility.

The difference between taking a seriously injured person to a regular emergency room and taking him to a Level I trauma center can be life or death. Statistics show that if you're seriously injured you have a 25 percent better chance of survival if you're taken directly to a Level I trauma center.

So in addition to getting the normal sort of maladies that would come into any ER—heart attacks, strokes, diabetic emergencies, gastrointestinal bleedings, cancer at the last stages, weird infections, babies being born—a hospital with a Level I trauma center gets the worst of the worst injury cases. And in an exciting and vibrant but also violent city like New Orleans, it was astonishing what you would see come through the doors at Charity Hospital.

Gunshot wounds, stabbings, bludgeonings, beatings, burnings, strangulations, falls, electrocutions, drownings, hangings, motorcycle accidents, car crashes. Every manner of violent injury that mishap or deadly intent can inflict on a human body came through the doors at Charity—and when they did, it was amazing to see how the trauma-team guys did their jobs. One minute everybody would be standing around, just routine, and then it would come over the PA system that a trauma red was coming in, and then the ER doors would fly open and the paramedics would wheel in some poor guy who was all bloody and broken and the doctors and residents and nurses would just descend on him, five or six of them, each with a specific job to do—one to manage the breathing and intubate, one to put in the IVs, one to put tubes into the chest if needed to draw away blood from internal bleeding, one cutting off the patient's clothes, one putting in a Foley catheter and doing a rectal exam, one cutting down on the ankles to get a vein, until they had the patient stabilized and ready for surgery if necessary. It looked like chaos, with blood and clothes and tubes flying all around, but in fact it was as carefully choreographed as a ballet.

It was also exciting, in a way that my previous medical train-

ing had not been. Sure, I had seen patients with cancer or conges-
tive heart failure or countless other life-threatening conditions,
and I had seen some of them die. But never before in my medical
training had I seen situations in which every second and every
decision could mean the difference between a patient living or
dying. It was an adrenaline rush.

Of course, as a med student, I was mostly just watching and
learning during those situations. At least at first, the medical students in the Charity ER—me and my USUHS buddy and the
others, mostly students from Tulane or LSU—generally did the
scut work, the minor stuff: suturing cuts, putting casts on broken
bones, getting test and lab results, treating scrapes and abrasions,
interviewing the walk-ins, people who just didn't feel well and
didn't have a doctor or insurance so they came into the ER.

A lot of them were ER regulars, known in medical terminol-
ogy as "frequent presenters" or, in slang, frequent flyers. They
were homeless people who checked into the ER to get a free meal
and a bed, or people with mental problems, drunks and drug
users or people who had chronic conditions and just needed a
little help. Sometimes it could get a little nasty. I remember this
one old lady who walked in complaining of stomach pain, and
she wasn't very lucid, and after trying to talk to her and examine
her my med-school buddy and I couldn't figure out what was
wrong with her. So we asked one of the interns, and he looked
over and recognized her and knew exactly what the problem was.
"Oh, yeah," he said. "Her. She's a regular. She's just impacted.
Go ahead and disimpact her." Which meant that while I held her
hand, my buddy, who had lost the coin toss, had to stick his finger up her butt and dislodge things a little bit, with her screaming, "Oh Lordy! Oh Lordy!" the whole time. And when he took
his finger out, well, it was an explosion of epic proportions. He
had to throw away his shoes after that.

Which is another thing to remember about ERs and trauma medicine in general. In America we like to think of medical care as clean, antiseptic, sterile—and in most medical fields it is. But especially in high-incident ERs and trauma centers like Charity, trauma and emergency medicine is full of shit, piss, vomit, blood, and BO, and all the Lysol in the world can never completely take the smell away. Trust me, if TV shows like *St. Elsewhere* or *ER* had been broadcast in Smell-o-Vision, hardly anybody would have been able to watch them. It's something you have to get used to, just like you have to get used to the sight of blood. If you aren't able to crack open a gunshot victim's chest and then fifteen minutes later sit down in the cafeteria and totally enjoy a slice of pepperoni pizza with extra red sauce, you'd better find another line of work. I said earlier that to be a trauma surgeon you have to put some Kevlar around your heart; I guess you also have to put some Kevlar around your stomach.

In any event, by the time I graduated from medical school in 1987, having experienced almost all of the medical special-ties during my various rotations, I had decided that I would be a surgeon. I guess it was my calling. I knew that the surgery route would be tough, and long, but it seemed like what I would be best at, and what I wanted to do—although I still didn't know that trauma surgery would turn out to be my specialty.

Since Uniformed Services University was a military institu-tion, the graduation ceremony itself was a spit-and-polish affair, with all of us marching around in our dress uniforms while our family members cheered. My mother and father came down for the ceremony and were very proud. It was held at the Kennedy Center, and the commencement speaker was President Ronald Reagan, who told us, "Yours is the only medical school in Amer-ica that trains physicians to be ready for duty on the bottom of the ocean or on the surface of the moon and any place in between." My parents were impressed. After graduation I moved up in rank from an ensign (O-1) to a Navy lieutenant (O-3), the equivalent of a captain in the other services, which was a nice jump in terms of pay and military status.

But I still had to do my surgery internship and then my residency. After all my training I would owe the taxpayers of the United States seven years of active duty service as a military doctor to pay them back for putting me through medical school. Then, I thought, I would go into private practice in whatever surgery specialty I had trained in—maybe general surgery, or maybe plastics, plastic surgery being the most lucrative and easygoing surgery specialty. I thought I had it all figured out—but of course I didn't.

I took my one-year surgery internship at the Naval Hospital San Diego, also known as Balboa Naval Hospital, a sprawling, red-tile-roofed complex next to Balboa Park in the heart of the city. The original Naval Hospital had been built in 1925, and in World War II it handled almost two hundred thousand casualties from the war in the Pacific Theater. During the Vietnam War it was the biggest military hospital in the world, again treating thousands of young Marines and sailors who had been seriously wounded in combat.

It was a good hospital, but by the time I got there, in practice it was a civilian hospital, in the sense that almost all of the medicine practiced there was not military oriented. Most of the patients were either retired military people or the dependent spouses and children of sailors and Marines, and the surgeries performed were the same as those on the civilian side: cancer, heart, orthopedic, and pediatric. There were no trauma cases to handle.

There was a reason for that. Military bases were then—and still are—just about the safest places in America to live and work.

Speed limits were fifteen miles per hour in populated areas, drunk driving wasn't tolerated, drug users were quickly discharged, there was virtually no crime, training exercises were closely regulated to prevent accidents. Most of the serious wounds or injuries suffered by military personnel happened off base—and in these cases, the victims were taken to civilian ERs or trauma centers.

So I never saw a trauma case—a shooting, a stabbing, a car accident—during my surgery internship. And the Navy didn't go out of its way to expose its surgeons-in-training to such things. After all, the Cold War was winding down, and with the tragedy of Vietnam still fresh in people's minds, no one expected the US to get involved in any major conflict in some far-flung corner of the world. The Navy decided that it needed surgeons who could cut a cancerous tumor out of a sixty-four-year-old retired chief petty officer, not surgeons who specialized in treating young Marines and sailors being carried off a medevac helicopter with their legs blown off or shrapnel in their brains.

I could understand the Navy medical command's argument that their budget didn't allow for trauma training for Navy doctors. But it bothered me that even though I was going to be a military doctor for the foreseeable future, I wasn't being trained for war. I was being trained for peace.

And eventually I realized that if I was ever going to learn how to be a doctor in wartime, I had to be where the real war was— that is, on America's urban streets.

CHAPTER 4

EMBRACING THE SUCK

I read somewhere that the first confirmed gunshot victim in the Western Hemisphere was an Inca Indian killed by a Spanish musket in the early 1500s. Archeologists excavating an ancient cemetery in Peru found the unfortunate man in 2004, his skeletal remains still showing the round, quarter-sized entry and exit holes in the skull that are consistent with a GSW—that is, a gunshot wound.

But if he was our hemisphere's first known GSW victim, it's an understatement to say he was hardly the last. In the five centuries since then, we've been gunning each other down with depressing regularity, and in numbers that are nothing short of astonishing.

The statistics vary from year to year, but according to the Centers for Disease Control and Prevention and other agencies, generally speaking there are about thirty thousand gun-related deaths in the US annually, including suicides, accidents, and homicides. A very small percentage of those gun homicides are legal—cops shooting a bad guy, a citizen defending himself. About nine thousand of them are out-and-out murders.

Of course, the would-be murderers don't always succeed. There are also about eighty thousand nonfatal gunshot injuries every year, about three quarters of them the result of interpersonal violence—one person shooting another.

The bottom line is that far more Americans are killed or wounded by gunfire in the US in a single year than the total number of American troops killed and wounded in a decade of wars in Iraq and Afghanistan.

Personally, I think we could reduce those numbers with some common-sense restrictions to help keep guns out of the hands of criminals and lunatics, without doing violence to the Second Amendment. At the very least, we should all keep in mind just how much our current policies on gun ownership are costing us—not just in terms of blood but in treasure as well. A gunshot wound doesn't just kill or wound one person; it wounds family members, friends, and society in general. And the public health costs for treating all those tens of thousands of gunshot victims are enormous. I can tell you from experience that a lot of gunshot victims don't have health insurance, which means that the taxpayers and people who do have insurance wind up paying the bill.

Of course, it's not just guns that kill and maim us. About two thousand people are stabbed or slashed to death every year, and another two thousand are beaten, strangled, asphyxiated, drowned, or otherwise slain at the hands of another. Traffic collisions claim in excess of thirty thousand lives every year and injure more than two million people. Another hundred thousand people die every year from falls, industrial accidents, drownings, electrocutions, and every other manner of mishap.

In all, about 150,000 people in America die of traumatic

injuries every year. For Americans under the age of twelve, the number-one cause of death is trauma. For Americans under eighteen, the number-one cause of death is trauma. For Americans under age forty-eight, the number-one cause of death is trauma. Not cancer, not heart disease. Trauma. Because it affects the young, trauma is the single greatest cause of years of life lost among Americans.

And yet only 10 percent of our national health care expenditures go to the treatment of traumatic injuries. Trauma research receives less than one tenth the amount of research money devoted to cancer, heart disease, and HIV.

Well, I could go on and on with the statistics, but you get the point. With all of those deaths and injuries, there is a critical need in America for trauma surgeons, for people trained in the distinct specialty of handling surgery and medical treatment in emergency situations.

The problem with trauma surgeons is that there just aren't that many doctors who are able, much less willing, to be one. Out of about 140,000 surgeons in the US, we have 36,000 OB-GYN surgeons, 20,000 orthopedic surgeons, 6,000 plastic surgeons—but only about 1,500 board-certified trauma surgeons.

It's a pretty small club. But after my first real exposure to trauma surgery, I began to realize that I didn't want to do anything else.

After my internship at Balboa hospital in San Diego, I had been scheduled to spend a three-year tour as a GMO (general medical officer) aboard a Navy oil tanker, a ship that resupplies fuel to other Navy ships while they're at sea. A GMO handles sick calls, hands out medicines, maintains the crew's medical records, treats minor injuries. If anything really serious comes up, the patient is, if possible, transferred shoreside or to a larger ship with more extensive medical staff and facilities.

I didn't really mind the prospect. After nine years of school and training, it would be a chance to get out on my own for a while and get some real-world experience. And after five years in the Navy I was ready for a little sea duty. Besides, the word was that the chow aboard the tankers was great.

Then fate intervened. My internship coordinator called me and congratulated me for being selected to go into a general surgery residency—which was interesting, since I hadn't applied for a general surgery residency. I was still thinking about plastic surgery. I figured there must have been some mistake. Then the chairman of surgery at the Navy's Graduate Medical Education Office, which handled all the Navy residencies, explained that the Navy needed more general surgeons in the pipeline—not for combat action, but for the kind of surgeries and maladies usually handled at Navy hospitals in peacetime: hernias, breast tumors, gallstones, appendicitis, pancreatitis, bowel obstructions, colon inflammation, cancer. So they were bending—actually breaking—the rules and selecting a candidate who would skip the GMO sea-duty requirement and go straight into a civilian general surgery residency. I was the top candidate, he said.

He made it sound like a good deal, but in fact there were some downsides. One was that since I would still be an active duty Navy officer and be paid by the Navy, I would owe the Navy eleven more years of active duty service after completing my medical training, instead of seven. When I asked the chairman if I could refuse, he said sure—but if I did it would seriously annoy members of the Navy medical brass who had gone to great lengths to get me this plum assignment.

Since I didn't have much of a choice, I decided to go for it. I started applying for civilian general surgery residency positions across the country, but there weren't many openings. Fortunately for me, one of the second-year residents at University of California Irvine Medical Center had quit, so they called me up for an interview. I drove from San Diego up to UCIMC, a modern, glass-and-granite complex surrounded by palm trees near the Santa Ana Freeway in northeastern Orange County. I walked in with my file bulging with glowing recommendations from everybody I had worked with, thinking that this interview was going to be a breeze.

But it wasn't. The chairman, Dr. Mason, sat me down at the end of a long boardroom conference table while he sat at the other end and started going through my file. Then he asked me what I wanted to do at UCI, and I barked out the preapproved, standard-issue Navy response, the answer the Navy had told me to give: "Sir, I want to be a good general surgeon!"

Wrong answer. Dr. Mason closed my file folder, put it on the table, and slid it all the way across to me like he didn't even want to touch it.

"Well, in that case we don't want you here," he said. "What we're looking for is an academic surgeon, someone who is going to further our field, who will improve our profession, who will do research and teach others. There are a lot of community training programs that will make you a good general surgeon. If that's all you want to be, you should look for a job elsewhere."

In other words, we don't want a guy who is only using our training as a stepping-stone to a nice life doing routine surgeries and pulling in a big paycheck and going home to the wife and kids at the same time every evening. We want a guy who's committed to the higher ideals of our profession, someone who will do research, write and defend papers, investigate new procedures and methods, someone who will question medical orthodoxy, someone who will make a difference.

I was dumbfounded. I mumbled something and fled the room, convinced that I had blown the opportunity. But at the same time, there was something about what Dr. Mason had said that struck me.

Until that time I had always thought of medicine as a career, not a calling. The truth is that I had been more concerned about what I could get out of being a doctor than in what I could put into being a doctor, what I could contribute to the profession of medicine. But Dr. Mason was right. Sooner or later I had to decide which kind of doctor I wanted to be—and eventually, as we'll see, I would realize that I didn't want to be just a good general surgeon.

Anyway, after the blown interview I called one of my medical-school mentors at USUHS, Dr. Norman Rich, a world-famous Vietnam War surgeon. I told him what had happened, and he told me not to worry about it, that he would call Dr. Mason. I don't know what he told him, but it worked. I got the job.

Well, I call it a job. But a surgical residency, especially back then, was actually more like a form of institutional slavery.

Under the general surgery residency program you went through rotations in all the various types of surgeries: surgical oncology, cardiothoracic, vascular, gastrointestinal, colorectal, urological, pediatric, transplant, and trauma/acute care. The idea was to give you a basic grounding in every kind of surgical procedure, and then eventually you would choose a particular specialty. Some of those rotations, such as plastics or urology, were easier than others. But overall, being a surgical resident, especially a junior one, was a backbreaking, brain-numbing grind.

Sure, you got to assist in all types of surgical procedures, and you learned a lot about the technical aspects of surgery. But the actual cutting was only a small part of it. The vast majority of your time was spent outside the operating room, checking on pre-op or post-op patients, seeing patients in clinic, reviewing lab tests, prescribing medications, writing up endless charts and histories and other paperwork. There were times as a junior resident when you might have fifty or sixty patients to attend to, many of them critically ill—and if you screwed up, you would hear about it from your bosses, who were constantly looking over your shoulder. A serious error, or a series of small ones, could get you dismissed from the residency program. It was a pyramid system. Every year someone would be cut from the program, so there was a lot of competition.

Even though this was in the civilian world, the residency system was as rigidly hierarchical as the military world. The attending physicians told the chief residents (the guys in their final year of residency) what to do, the chief residents told the senior residents (the guys in their third and fourth years) what to do, the senior residents told the junior residents (guys in their first and second years) what to do, and the junior residents got to tell the interns what to do. And the same inalterable principle of physics that applied in the military also ruled in the civilian residency world—that is, the crap always rolled downhill. The more of his overwhelming workload a senior resident could pass down to a junior resident, the more able he was to finish the overwhelming workload that had been passed down to him by a chief resident. And so on.

The upshot was that in an average week, the other residents and I would put in 100 to 120 hours at the hospital, and some weeks 140 hours or more—and, remember, an entire seven-day week has only 168 hours in it. In fact, the term *resident* derives from the fact that in the old days, doctors in training actually lived—resided—in the hospital. And we came pretty close to doing that. We all had places to live, but we rarely saw them. There was an intern I worked with who slept in his car in the hospital parking lot whenever he got a few hours off, and shaved and showered in the hospital call rooms before reporting for work. He said he was so tired that he didn't feel safe going home and would rather use the driving time to get more sleep. In other words, this future doctor in training was technically a homeless guy.

As you can imagine, when you're working 120 hours or more a week, sleep becomes the most important thing in the world to you—more important than food, which you generally get out of a vending machine anyway. You simply can't get enough sleep. You can try to grab an hour or two while you're on call, but chances are you'll barely close your eyes before you get a call, for anything ranging from a patient coding in the ICU to a nurse who has a medication question. When this goes on for week after week, you often find yourself in a semicomatose state; there were times when I would be driving home for a few hours' sleep after working forty straight hours and I'd be jarred back to consciousness by the thump-thump-thump-thump of my car tires hitting the raised reflective markers separating the lanes, a phenomenon known in California as "driving by Braille." Sometimes I wondered if we residents were actually human lab rats in some elaborate secret government study on the effects of long-term sleep deprivation. I wondered, too, if anybody other than my surgery colleagues really understood the slavelike apprenticeships that surgeons have to go through.

It's different these days. The medical accreditation agencies, concerned about the effects of fatigue on medical care, have begun limiting residents' work weeks to no more than eighty hours. I think it's the right thing to do—I don't believe in exhausted residents—but it has also caused a host of problems. With their hours limited, surgical residents are coming out of hospitals without the necessary experience; they simply haven't put in enough hours to learn all the things they need to learn. To fix that, the residency requirement for surgeons is being changed to seven years instead of five. Meanwhile, attending physicians have had to fill the void, spending countless extra hours doing the work that residents used to do—and I don't believe in exhausted attendings, either. Ultimately we're going to have to develop a system in which doctors work fewer hours, even if it means they make less money.

In any event, the long hours as a resident might not have been quite so bad if the paychecks hadn't been so pathetic. Even though I was working on the civilian side, the Navy was paying my salary—as a lieutenant, about $30,000 a year. That would have been okay for a regular job, but not for the kind of hours I was working. I figured out that during my second year of residency I worked almost six thousand hours. Thirty thousand dollars divided by six thousand hours equals five bucks an hour—at the time, minimum wage.

Of course, not everybody made it through the surgical residency program. Every year the number of residents got smaller as some people who didn't make the grade were let go, while others, beaten down by the long hours and heavy workload, simply quit and went into some other, easier medical field.

And despite the long hours and the hard work, I knew that at the end there would be a payoff. When I started, I figured I would complete my five-year general surgery residency, do a fellowship in a surgical subspecialty—say, for example, plastic surgery— finish up my Navy obligation, and then go into private practice and live a nice, safe, easy, and extremely lucrative life doing nose jobs and breast augmentations. I might even take up golf.

So even though I bitched about the long hours like everybody else, I got through them. I was twenty-seven years old when I started at UCI, physically in great shape, and while I was as tired and sleep-deprived as everybody else, I never even thought about quitting.

And I discovered I was good at it—not just the cutting part of being a surgeon, but the patient-care part as well. In my training program, much of my time as a surgical resident was spent in the ICU, taking care of critically ill people. I found that I had kind of a sixth sense about what was going on with them; I could sense when they were going to have problems. It seemed like whenever a patient in the ICU "coded"—that is, went into cardiopulmonary arrest—I was there, and I knew what to do about it. I had a knack for being in the right place at the right time.

But while I found myself being drawn toward the excitement and action of critical care, I still wasn't thinking about being a trauma surgeon. That changed on the first day of my first clinical rotation, when I had to take a dead woman's heart in my hands—literally.

Orange County had long enjoyed a reputation for being one of the safest places to live in California, a quiet, orderly, planned-community refuge for people fleeing the urban ills of Los Angeles. And for a while that was an accurate depiction. But gangs, drugs, and violence pay no attention to county borders. By the time I got there in 1988, the violent reality of life in LA had started to seep into the OC. The UCI Trauma Center, the only Level I trauma center in the county, was handling hundreds of gunshot wounds, stabbings, beatings, and assorted other cases of person-on-person mayhem every year. And within an hour after I reported for duty in my first rotation in the trauma center, another victim of that mayhem came rolling through the swinging doors.

She was in her late fifties, somebody's mother or grandmother. She was not a player in the deadly games being acted out in the streets of Anaheim and Santa Ana and Garden Grove, but instead just an innocent bystander to a gang shooting who had happened to catch a bullet in the chest that had been intended for someone else—although it often seemed as if the gangsters really didn't care whom they shot, as long as they could shoot someone. She had coded in the ambulance on the way to the trauma center, five minutes before they wheeled her in—"coded" meaning that she had died, in the sense that she had stopped breathing and her heart had stopped beating. The EMTs in the ambulance had been giving her CPR, but her heart hadn't started beating when they brought her into the trauma bay.

So the trauma team's first job was to bring her back from the dead. And the only way to do that was to perform a resuscitative thoracotomy, which is another way of saying that we had to cut open her chest to massage her heart. And we had to do it fast, because every second she was dead increased the chances she would stay that way.

As an intern and junior resident I had already assisted in scores of surgical procedures. But those had all taken place in the quiet, sterile, orderly confines of an operating room, where you basically had all the time in the world. I had never had to perform a major surgical procedure in the controlled chaos of a trauma bay, where every second counted. Before I had even reported for my trauma rotation I had studied up on the necessary protocols and guidelines, so intellectually I knew what to do, but I had never actually had to do it before. Still, when the senior resident who was in charge of the trauma team said we were going to do a resuscitative thoracotomy and told me to start cutting, I knew I couldn't hesitate.

I was terrified.

It's a funny thing about being scared. Some people fall completely apart when they're afraid: the pitch of their voice rises, their hands shake, their judgment gets muddled, and they doubt their own decisions. With other people, fear focuses them, concentrates them, empowers them. Their hands are steady, their voices are calm and even, they seem to know exactly what to do;

they understand that the point is not to have no fear, but to not show that fear. Maybe it was my military background, my time in the field with the Marines, or maybe it was just the luck of the draw. But I was in the latter group.

So after the nurses splashed a topical antiseptic all over the woman's chest, I took a scalpel and quickly and confidently started cutting. I cut through her skin from her sternum and under her left breast and all the way to the back, which exposes the chest wall. Ordinarily at that point you have to cut through the muscles that hold the ribs together. But my adrenaline was kicking in, so instead I just used my hands to spread the ribs apart so we could put in the Finochietto rib spreader to get access to the heart. Then I grabbed her silent heart with both hands.

The purpose of open-chest cardiac massage is to have your hands do the work the victim's heart usually does—that is, pump blood out, particularly to the brain, and then suck it back into the heart. Doing CPR through the chest on a patient who has no blood in the heart is useless; that's why you have to do open-heart massage. Nothing else will save her.

So once you open her up, you put a clamp on the aorta to keep the blood from flowing to the lower half of the body, where it's not needed as much as it's needed in the brain and heart. Meanwhile another set of surgeons puts a tube into the trachea to get air into the lungs. So as you squeeze the heart you're pumping oxygenated blood to the brain and back to the vessels that feed the heart, and when you release it, the oxygenated blood flows back into the heart; without that oxygenated blood, the brain and heart will die within minutes.

It's a fast and physically demanding process; you're doing about seventy or ninety compressions per minute. At the same time, you take a syringe with epinephrine in it and you inject it directly into the left ventricle chamber to get the maximum effect. Then you go back to doing the open-heart massage. If it doesn't work, you try shocking the heart with internal defibrillator paddles that are placed directly onto the heart to give it a kick start. At the same time, you're looking for the damage caused by the bullet, and clamping off any damaged arteries that are bleeding. In this particular case, the dead woman had been shot in the center of the vessels that feed the lungs. The hope is that you can get the heart beating again, that she will come back to life, and then you can send her to the operating room, where the damage can be repaired.

Unfortunately, it's a slim hope. If you're alive when you're brought into a Level I trauma center, you have on average a 95 percent chance of surviving, at least in the short term. Depending on the severity of your injuries, postoperative complications may claim your life, but generally speaking, if you come into the trauma center alive you'll leave the trauma center alive. But if you come into the trauma center already dead, your chances plummet dramatically. In cases requiring trauma-related thoracotomies, only about one in twenty—5 percent—comes back to life.

This woman wasn't that one out of twenty. The damage to her lungs was too great; she had already been dead too long. After ten minutes of squeezing her heart we had to give up, and the senior resident "pronounced" her—that is, declared her dead. She came to us dead on arrival—DOA—and she would stay that way.

As an intern and a surgical resident I had already seen a lot of people die. Still, you can't remain completely immune to the grief that death, particularly sudden, unexpected death, inevitably brings with it. Even though this poor woman was a complete stranger, I felt sad that her life had been stolen from her.

Yet at the same time I also felt—well, exhilarated by my work.

That may sound strange, but when the trauma center doors burst open and a person with life-threatening injury is wheeled in, there's no time for cautious deliberation, for slowly weighing pros and cons, for consulting the literature and examining the protocols; a lot of times they don't even have a protocol for what you're faced with. You have to act, right now, right this second—and for me there was no greater adrenaline rush than in taking quick action.

There was also the fact that never before in my professional life had I felt quite so vital, so necessary as when I was holding that woman's heart in my hands. Sure, a person with a cancerous tumor needs an oncological surgeon, and a person with a hernia needs a general surgeon, and even a person with a less than perfect nose needs a plastic surgeon, or thinks he does. But I submit that no one in the world needs someone quite as desperately and immediately as a person dying from a bullet in the chest needs a trauma surgeon.

Then, too, there was the realization that after six years in the military as a student and an intern and a junior resident, this was the first time I had been personally involved in treating someone with a gunshot wound or any other kind of penetrating traumatic injury—which was exactly the kind of injury that young soldiers, Marines, sailors, and airmen would suffer if we ever got into a war. I was a Navy officer, and would be for the foreseeable future as I fulfilled my military commitment. So it seemed to me that the Navy didn't need more doctors who specialized in neonatology or rheumatology. It needed more doctors who had been specifically trained in how to save young men and women with broken and torn bodies.

(In fact, that shortage of military trauma specialists would become apparent during the Persian Gulf War in 1991—a war that to my intense frustration I was forced to miss because I was still in my residency. More than twenty thousand active duty and reserve doctors, nurses, medics, corpsmen, and other medical personnel were deployed in that conflict, but only a handful of the surgeons were trauma specialists. That could have posed a serious problem if, as initially predicted, US forces had suffered tens of thousands of casualties requiring emergency surgery. Fortunately, as it turned out, there were only 147 US battle deaths and 467 wounded personnel—bad enough, but not nearly as bad as it could have been.)

Of course, the people you work with and admire also play a big role in your direction in life. Dr. Ken Waxman, a trauma surgeon who was director of critical care at UCI, was a major influence in my decision to go into trauma. He wasn't the smoothest guy socially—a bit gruff and brusque—and if you needed hand-holding, he wasn't your guy. But if you were sick, injured, or dying, you couldn't have asked for anybody better. He had a reputation among the residents as being the smartest guy in the hospital, and if his hands were a little rough, surgically speaking, he more than made up for it in smarts. He was a small man physically, but he cast a huge shadow. I admired him a lot.

The chief resident in the UCI trauma unit, Dr. Gail Tominaga, was another big influence on me. Smart, straightforward, thoroughly capable, what impressed me about her was her thoroughness, her attention to detail. While other residents making the rounds in the ICU might jot down a few notes for the nurses to follow in a patient's care, Dr. Tominaga would write pages. She didn't miss a thing. It was a quality I would try to emulate in my own career.

In any event, as I went through my trauma and critical-care rotations it became increasingly clear to me that that was what I wanted to do, a feeling that only grew as my general surgery residency continued.

I had other options. For example, the doctors in cardiothoracic and heart transplant surgery were recruiting me heavily to go into their field. One of my favorites was Dr. Richard Ott, head of the UCI heart transplant program. He kept trying to set me up with his friend "Jack in Arizona" for a few years' training after my residency. It turned out that "Jack" was Dr. Jack Copeland, a nationally renowned heart transplant surgeon and pioneer in the development of the total artificial heart who was head of the transplant program at University of Arizona Medical Center in Tucson. Of course, later I would wind up in Tucson—but not in heart transplants.

But despite the other opportunities, at the time nothing else seemed to offer the excitement and personal satisfaction of trauma and critical care. As a trauma surgeon I wouldn't be spending my life taking out gall bladders or fixing hernias and doing the same procedures all day long. Every case would be different, and I would get to work in almost every aspect of surgery, from vascular to cardiothoracic to neurosurgery and on and on. Whatever came through the doors, I would have to know how to handle it.

I knew there would be downsides to it. Those one-hundred-plus-hour weeks I was putting in as a resident would continue as a trauma surgeon. I knew I would pretty much have to give up Friday and Saturday nights, that I would be almost constantly on duty or on call, that it wouldn't leave room for much of a home life. I knew too that as a trauma surgeon I would never make as much money as a cardiothoracic surgeon, much less a plastics guy. I knew full well that being a trauma surgeon is one of the toughest, most physically demanding jobs a surgeon can have.

But I guess that was a big part of what drew me to it. In the military there's a phrase people use about doing the hard thing, the challenging thing, the thing that most people can't or won't do, and doing it without whining or complaining. It's called "embracing the suck."

I knew that as a trauma surgeon, I would be embracing the suck.

Anyway, in my third year of residency I let it be known that I was going to specialize in trauma/critical care. It wasn't a formal announcement or anything; the word just kind of got around. It was sort of like joining a fraternity, a brotherhood and sisterhood. All of the other trauma people, like Dr. Waxman and Dr. Tominaga and others, started treating me differently, giving me more responsibility, taking more time to teach me what they knew. If you're a trauma specialist and you've got a resident working for you who you know isn't interested in going into trauma, who's just trying to make it through the rotation, well, you naturally aren't as interested in spending time with him or her, teaching him or her, as you are with somebody who's going to do trauma for a career.

Even the ICU nurses started treating me differently when they found out that I was going to specialize in trauma and acute care, that I was joining their club. If they had a patient crashing they would always call me, and they went out of their way to help me gain from their experiences. Unfortunately, a lot of young doctors treat nurses like the hired help and don't really value their opinions, which to me is just stupid. Some of those ICU nurses were taking care of critically ill patients when the young doctor on call was still in elementary school, and while the doctor is in charge, often the only way to truly know what's going on with a patient is to listen to the nurse.

The fact is that I have a soft spot for nurses. As a general rule I think they're some of the most dedicated, selfless, compassionate people I know.

And I'm not just saying that because I married one.

I know, it's kind of a cliché, a doctor marrying a nurse and vice versa. But when you're working 120 hours a week in a hospital, who are you going to meet? You're going to meet other people who work in the hospital. I met Emily during my chief year, my fifth year of residency, shortly after she started as a night-shift nurse in the ICU. We actually met over an ICU patient who was coding, and while I was a little busy at the time, I wasn't too busy to notice that this nurse was not only smart and extremely competent but also a knockout. For reasons I'll never fully understand, she seemed to be a little impressed with me as well. One thing led to another, and pretty soon we were engaged.

There was, however, one potential problem in our relationship, one of the oldest problems in the history of romance—that is, her father. Emily's parents were both French-Canadian by birth, and her father, who worked as a facilities manager for a school district in the Orange County community of Placentia, was a pretty traditional, old-school kind of guy. The idea that his daughter was going to marry someone not of the Caucasian persuasion did not exactly fill him with enthusiasm.

But the Navy saved me. When he was just sixteen, Emily's dad, who was known as Frenchie, had lied about his age and joined the US Navy, putting in twenty years and retiring as a chief petty officer before taking the school district job. And he was still Navy, still sporting a Navy haircut, still maintaining a perfect Navy "gig line" in his clothes. So while the fact that I was a doctor didn't impress him, the fact that I was an active duty lieutenant commander with eight years in the Navy did. Even though he was an old salty dog and I hadn't yet done any sea duty, we had something in common. He decided that as a Navy officer, I would be a suitable son-in-law.

Besides, the sea-duty thing was coming soon enough. During my chief resident year I had applied for a fellowship in surgical critical care, critical care (also called intensive care) being a relatively new medical specialty at the time. Historically, surgeons had maintained control of their patients during the post-op recovery phase, but more and more that job of caring for critically ill patients after surgery was being handed over to board-certified critical-care specialists, known as "intensivists." As a trauma surgeon I didn't want to just patch up injured people and then pass them off to another doctor in the ICU. I wanted to be the captain of the patients' ship, so to speak, to be in charge of their treatment from the time they came into the trauma center until, ideally, they left the hospital. A fellowship and board certification in critical-care medicine would allow me to do that.

That was all fine with the Navy. But first, after nine years as a Naval officer, I finally had to go to sea.

I was assigned to a one-year tour as a surgeon aboard the USS *Carl Vinson*, a nuclear-powered aircraft carrier that at the time was just getting out of a dry-dock refit in Puget Sound Navy Yard in Bremerton, Washington. Carriers operate on a three-year cycle: a year of refit in dry dock, a year of workups or "sea trials" to make sure everything is functioning smoothly, and then a year's deployment as the centerpiece of a carrier battle group, which includes a dozen or so cruisers, destroyers, submarines, and other ships. I caught the *Vinson* just as it was starting its workups. The ship would go out for a day on Puget Sound, just to make sure it would still float, then out to sea for a few days, then for a couple of weeks. It was like a combination of shore duty and sea duty.

The *Vinson* had an extensive medical staff: a senior medical officer who was in charge, a general medical officer (GMO), a surgeon—me—and about fifty corpsmen and medical techs. We were responsible for the everyday medical needs of the *Vinson*'s five-thousand-man crew (female sailors weren't assigned to combatant Navy ships until later that year) as well as any medical situations the GMOs aboard the battle-group support ships couldn't handle on their own.

It was sort of like being a small-town doctor, except that almost all of our patients were young and in good physical shape. You'd have the usual colds, flu, urinary tract infections, minor scrapes and sprains, but the medical part usually wasn't too demanding. The biggest problem we had was seasickness; every time the ship would go out to sea we'd have a couple hundred guys lined up at sick bay the first day, all throwing up. But eventually they got used to it.

Still, you can't put five thousand guys on a rolling, pitching platform full of dangerous machinery without some accidents. Fingers would get caught in slamming hatches, guys would fall down gangways and break bones, flight deck crewmen would get too close to a jet intake. Occasionally we had to do some urgent surgeries, which were a little different from those in the civilian world. I remember once we had a young sailor who needed an emergency appendectomy, so the captain had to turn into the wind, slow to minimum speed, and cease all air operations in order to ease the ship's movement while we were cutting. Civilian surgeons seldom have to deal with an OR that's pitching and rolling. Later the captain came on the overhead speaker and announced throughout the ship that thanks to the valorous efforts of the medical staff the patient had survived and normal operations could resume, which we on the medical staff thought was pretty funny. For us, if not for the young sailor, the operation had been strictly routine.

But if the medical side was relatively easy, the Navy side wasn't. It wasn't like we were lounging around in deck chairs or anything. We spent hours and hours on drills, practicing how to handle mass casualties, how to get them to the sick bay, what to do if there's an electrical blackout or smoke or fire, whatever.

I'd have to write out the standard operating procedure for every eventuality you could imagine, and to do that I had to learn every passageway and bulkhead and hatch on the ship—which isn't easy on a ship that's more than three football fields long. Also, I wanted to get my Surface Warfare Officer pin, which is the first step in eventually getting command of a ship—even though as a doctor that wasn't going to be my career path. But I wanted that pin, so I had to learn about navigation, propulsion, nuclear reactors, how the catapults operated, the capabilities of every piece of ordnance on an F-18, and on and on. It was great fun—and for the first time, I really felt like I was a Navy officer.

Meanwhile, as I was beginning my *Vinson* tour, Emily and I had gotten married. My mom and dad came out, and Emily's mom and dad, and Emily wore a beautiful white dress and I put on my Navy dress whites and the *Vinson*'s chaplain married us right there at the Navy Yard. Emily and I rented a little one-bedroom cabin in the woods right on the water in Oyster Bay, and it was like paradise, one of those times you look back on and wish it could have gone on forever.

We also started making a family. Our son, Michael, was born after I finished the *Vinson* tour, as I was starting my fellowship in trauma and critical care at the University of Washington/ Harborview Medical Center in Seattle. Later, in 2000, we were blessed with our daughter, Anna. They were and are both great kids, although looking back on it, one of my great regrets is that I wasn't able to spend as much time with them as I wanted to.

But I couldn't. In June 1995, I completed my fellowship and became a certified trauma surgeon, with all the long hours and lack of home life that entails. As I said earlier, some people work to live, but trauma surgeons live to work. And there was a lot of work to be done.

For the next almost twenty years after completing my surgical training, and continuing to this day, I would practice my profession in some of the busiest and bloodiest trauma centers in America. Since my retirement from the Navy I've been a civilian trauma surgeon in Tucson, but before that I was an active duty Navy officer working and gaining experience in the civilian world while also being periodically deployed at sea and overseas in Iraq and Afghanistan. In 1994 and 1995 I was a clinical instructor and fellow at Harborview Medical Center in Seattle; from 1995 to 2000 I was an attending surgeon and Navy liaison officer at Washington Hospital Center in Washington, DC, and from 2002 to 2007 I was an attending trauma surgeon at Los Angeles County–University of Southern California Medical Center (known as County-USC) in LA. During that time I performed thousands of emergency surgeries, sometimes as many as a dozen a day. And while I remember the cases that were particularly challenging and interesting medically, the truth is that with most of the adult patients I've treated, I can't really remember all their faces.

But then there were some, too many of them, whose faces I wish I could forget.

CHAPTER 5

THE TRAUMA LIFE

The little kids are always the worst. The bullet holes look so big in their tiny bodies.

I remember one in particular, a little six-year-old girl who'd made the mistake of being asleep in her bed one night while grown-ups with guns were playing their murderous games. A car had rolled slowly past the little girl's house and two guys inside had opened up with 9-millimeter handguns, an apparent attempt to exact some sort of street-gang justice on one of the little girl's older brothers. They missed the brother clean, but one of the bullets had gone through the thin wall of the house like it was tissue paper and hit the sleeping little girl in the belly.

It's hard to say whether she was dead or not by the time the EMTs got to her; they could feel only a hint of a pulse. They packed her into the ambulance and inserted a pediatric-size endotracheal tube into her throat and started bag ventilating her, forcing air in and out of her lungs, while also performing chest compressions to try to get her heart beating. She wasn't responding. But even if she had responded, the fact is that all the CPR in the world can't save you if you're bleeding to death internally. For that you need a trauma surgeon who can go in and make the bleeding stop.

And it's not a case where every minute counts. It's a case where every second counts. By the time they brought her, lights flashing and siren screaming, to the trauma center, twelve minutes had passed since the EMTs had gotten to the little girl.

Although we have special pediatric-size instruments and devices we use on children, the initial procedure when they're rolled in through the trauma center doors is the same as for adults. My trauma team of residents and nurses and techs swarmed over her, one at the neck, one at the groin, one at the wrist, all feeling for a pulse, the respiratory tech at the head, others putting in IVs and pressure cuffs, another cutting away her blood-soaked pink pajamas with surgical scissors until she was completely nude. This all happened simultaneously, in a matter of seconds.

Again, with a child it seems different than with an adult, a question of scale. All those hands seem so big, and the body so small.

One by one the nurses and residents at the neck, groin, and wrist called out, "No pulse!" "No pulse!" "No pulse!" Protocol holds that a patient with penetrating trauma who hasn't responded after fifteen minutes of CPR is dead, and this little girl was now near that limit. But you never know. Sometimes the reported nonresponsive time is wrong. And kids are actually more resilient; they can be brought back to life more often than adults. So with a little child, you have to try. With a little child, everyone—nurses, techs, residents, cops, EMTs, yourself—expects you to try.

"Open her," I said. They all knew what I meant and they all knew what to do. One of the nurses splashed antiseptic Betadine over her chest and I took a scalpel and quickly cut laterally along the left side of her chest, from the breastbone all the way around to her back. I plunged my hands in between the ribs and spread them, then held them open with a child-size retractor. A quick look told me that the bullet had done extensive damage in her belly. I put a vascular clamp on the aorta above the injury in the chest to shut off blood flow to all but the heart and brain. We injected epinephrine directly into her left ventricle to stimulate her heart, and I took her heart in my hands and started massaging it, trying to get it to start beating.

Her heart was so small in my hands. The others were frantically getting a line into her veins and starting to give her warmed blood, while the chief resident was putting a tube into her right chest to see if there was any blood on that side, and in case the lung had collapsed in her right chest. After less than thirty seconds I stopped to look at her heart. It had started to beat, but slowly. We injected another small dose of epinephrine into her heart and I went back to massaging it. Another thirty seconds, and then her heart was beating strongly on its own. I looked up and said, "We've got her back. Let's go!"

I looked outside the trauma bay and saw the operating room nurse standing at the entry, waiting. I gave her a nod, and she instantly knew what that meant. It meant that we were taking the little girl to the OR that was reserved for me, that there was still a chance. She ran ahead to alert the OR team that we were coming, and fast. The nurses unlocked the little girl's trauma room bed and we started running to the OR, pushing the bed along; blood was dripping off the bed and leaving a trail on the floor behind us.

Seconds later the OR doors swung open, and we basically threw the little girl onto the OR table; there wasn't time to be gentle. The medical students on call that night had been running along with us and they crowded into the operating room as well, mouths agape, stunned at what they were seeing—so stunned, in fact, that they had forgotten they were in the OR, and they needed to put caps and masks on. The OR nurse was having none of it. "Get out and put masks on!" she yelled at them and they sheepishly backed out. They would learn.

The surgical residents and I were already capped and masked, and we walked into the surgical gowns the techs were holding up for us; the nurse tied up the backs as we put our gloves on. We hadn't scrubbed our hands because there just wasn't time. At the moment, infection was the last of our worries. We could take care of any potential infection later—if the little girl survived.

We moved to the operating room table, quickly threw a sterile drape on the child, and within seconds the scalpel was running down the little girl's abdomen, cutting through skin, fascia, and muscle in three long, sure, purposeful swipes. The residents know that in trauma we have to get in there fast, and that's the way I teach them to do it; there's no time for cautious maneuvering. Her abdomen was full of blood, so we started packing in surgical sponges to absorb it so we could get an idea of where the blood was coming from.

There are basically four stages to trauma surgery. The first is to stop the bleeding, the second is to control contamination, the third is to determine the extent of the injuries, and the last is to reconstruct the damaged parts. I could see that the little girl was bleeding from her main artery to the intestines. There was no way that this was going to be good. She also had numerous holes in her intestines, and her liver was bleeding from two holes made by the one bullet.

I quickly got a clamp on the major bleeder. This was really bad. If I couldn't stop the bleeding and then reconstruct the artery, she wouldn't have any blood supply to her entire small intestine, in which case the tissue would start to die. Even if she survived, that could make her life miserable, as she might never be able to eat and digest normally.

Just when the clamps were on, the anesthesiologist called out that the little girl no longer had a pulse. I abandoned my efforts in her abdomen and looked into her still-open chest to see what her heart was doing. It was giving out and slowing down.

"More freaking blood! Now!" I loudly called out.

"We're already giving her everything we have!" the anesthesiologist yelled back. There was a delay in getting more blood from the blood bank.

I started massaging her heart again, and again she came back. I moved back into her abdomen and started trying to stop the bleeding from her liver. Suddenly the anesthesiologist called out, "She's going down again!" So I went back into her chest and brought her back and then went back to her abdomen, only to have her heart start failing again. Chest, abdomen, chest, abdomen—the back and forth seemed to go on forever, but actually it was only about thirty minutes.

But finally it was too much for her. The anesthesiologist said, "Dr. Rhee, she's gone. She's gone. We don't have a pulse." But still I kept trying. Finally I came to my senses and looked around. Everyone was quiet and looking at me. I realized that it was hopeless.

"I'm going to stop," I told them. "Does anyone in this room have any other suggestions?" Everyone shook their heads no. I looked up at the clock and announced the official time of death— 0240 hours. I pulled down the sterile barrier between me and the anesthesiologist and then looked at the little girl's face.

I wish I could say she looked peaceful lying there on the OR table, but she didn't. Her eyes were wide open and lifeless, her mouth agape. She had a tube down her throat, she was covered in blood and Betadine, and in an effort to try to bring her back to life we had had to tear her small body apart. Maybe later, at her funeral, with the help of the undertaker's art, she would look peaceful, wearing a pretty pink dress, her eyes closed, her little hands crossed over her chest. But not now. Not now.

"We are all very sorry," I said to her. "We all tried, but we can't help you. Good night, go in peace."

I always apologize to patients who die, even though I know they can't hear me. But then, who's to say? Maybe in some way they can.

I left the room as the residents started closing the incisions and the nurses started getting the body ready for the medical examiner. There was blood all over me, so I had to change my scrubs and hose off my shoes. I wear waterproof red gardening shoes when I'm working so the bloodstains aren't so obvious. And as I was washing my hands at the scrub sink outside the OR, something happened that hadn't happened before.

I started crying.

Maybe it was because my own daughter was the same age as the little girl who had just died. Maybe it was the unfairness of this little girl being born in a place and a circumstance where a bullet could find her while she was sleeping. Maybe it was because I was so terribly tired. Whatever the reason, I found myself standing at the sink, sobbing uncontrollably.

And then as quickly as it came, it passed. I looked around and saw that fortunately, I was alone. No one had seen me break down. They can't see me break down. If the leader breaks down the troops will lose confidence in him, and it may cause them to break down as well. We simply don't have time for that.

I washed my face and headed to the locker room.

Of course, the six-year-old who died that night wasn't the first badly injured child I'd had to deal with, or the last. In fact, incredibly, earlier that very same evening we had another young girl come in with a gunshot wound—although in that case we couldn't even try to save her. She had been shot in the head and the back of her head was blown open and her brain was hanging out.

It's a horrible thing to see a young child like that—and I have seen it far too many times. And yet part of me wishes that everyone in America would have to see what I have seen. If people had to see those little children as I and other trauma surgeons and trauma center personnel have to see them, lying bloody and torn up in a trauma bay, I know that we as a nation would do more to try to stop it.

The numbers are appalling. In 2010 there were 172 children under the age of twelve who were shot and killed by firearms in the US. That's equal to almost nine Sandy Hook Elementary School child massacres, but because they happen in ones or twos, they usually don't rate much more than a single story in the newspaper, or a few minutes on the local TV news. Meanwhile, thousands more young children are wounded by guns, not to mention being stabbed, beaten, and otherwise abused by adults.

It's hard enough to deal with a child who comes in with a sudden traumatic injury. It's even worse when a little one- or two-year-old kid comes in unconscious with a head injury and you see a bunch of old bruises on his body. You do a full workup on cases like that, X-raying every bone in their bodies, and every time that film pops up and you see an old, untreated healing fracture you picture that poor little kid being beaten and beaten and beaten until finally he gets one hit too many, one hit too hard, and he never wakes up. It breaks your heart, and it fills you with rage against anyone who could do that to a helpless child.

I said before that to be a trauma surgeon you have to put some Kevlar around your heart. But the little kids are the chink in the Kevlar.

It's not that I don't feel sympathy for adult trauma victims as well. I've dealt with hundreds of innocent adult victims who wound up in a trauma bay with bullet and knife wounds through absolutely no fault of their own: a University of Arizona dance student hit by a stray AK-47 bullet from a gang shoot-out; a Korean mom-and-pop grocery store owner shot in the face by a robber after he'd already handed over the money; a dozen people shot and wounded just because they had wanted to shake hands with their congresswoman. In other cases the victims are otherwise law-abiding people who through momentary passion or too much alcohol—often both—find themselves in violent or dangerous situations: the truck driver who gets in an argument with his cousin over Thanksgiving dinner and winds up with a carving knife in his chest, or the lawyer who's arguing with his wife and catches a slug from the pistol he bought for "home protection." The list is endless.

But it's also a fact of life in the trauma business that a lot of our patients are willing players in the violent world they help create—gangbangers shot by other gangbangers, drug dealers shot by competitors, killers and armed robbers shot by cops. Maybe some of them are just born bad to the bone, while others are simply the products of the wrong environment. But either way they are participants in their own destruction.

It doesn't mean that we treat them any different medically. People sometimes wonder if I really try as hard to save a wounded armed robber as I would to save a wounded cop. The answer is yes. If as a trauma surgeon I start making moral judgments about the relative worth of my patients, I'm not doing my job. It's not our job to be judge and jury. And in trauma cases, if we give them anything less than the best care possible, we could wind up being executioners.

I remember one case, on a really busy Saturday night, with half a dozen seriously injured red blankets in the trauma bays— "red blankets" being the term for the heavy bleeders, which goes

82

back to the days when hospitals used red blankets instead of white sheets so the blood wouldn't show so much. Patients were screaming, people were yelling, nurses and techs were running around, EMTs and cops were everywhere—the usual Saturday-night pandemonium. It was just the sort of atmosphere in which stories can get mixed up.

I had this one guy opened up in the OR who had taken a bullet in the back. Someone said that he had shot a cop and then had been shot down by other cops. Whatever he was, he was bleeding badly from his vena cava in the right chest. I got my hand on it but I couldn't control it; it was hard to reach, under the diaphragm. This guy was going to die on me, as I couldn't seem to get control of his bleeding. So I called my backup surgeon at home to come in and give me a hand while I stood there with my fingers in the dike. Twenty-five minutes later he showed up, scrubbed in, then took a sucker tube that is used to draw away accumulated blood and started to look around.

"What happened to this guy?" he asked me. I shrugged and said, "I don't know. Something about shooting a cop."

To me it was just making conversation. It didn't matter how or why the guy got shot. But then, unbelievably, the backup surgeon took the sucker and put it on the torn vessel and started to suck out the blood. The guy was already bleeding to death, and now my backup was sucking his blood out even faster.

"What the hell are you doing?" I said. The surgeon looked at me like it was no big deal and said, "He killed a cop, right?"

I grabbed the sucker out of his hand and I said, "I don't know what he did. Are you gonna help me or not?" Finally he agreed to do his job, and while he held back the tissue I managed to get a suture and three throws of a stitch on the vein and the wounded guy finally stopped bleeding. When we were finished the backup surgeon walked away without a word. The wounded guy survived.

And as it turned out, the story on him had been completely wrong. Amid all the excited chatter in the trauma bays, the facts had gotten twisted around. The wounded guy hadn't shot a cop. Instead, he was a regular working stiff who'd been accidentally shot by a cop who was responding to a rape call and went to the wrong house. It was a major screwup on the cop's part—and on my backup surgeon's. I don't know if he had intentionally tried to ace the wounded guy by putting that sucker on a bleeding vein—I couldn't prove it—or if he was just being sloppy. But either way he had let his personal feelings and emotions override his medical ethics and responsibilities. Before that happened, I had always respected him for his surgical skills. Afterward, I couldn't respect him anymore.

Of course, while it doesn't give them the right to act on it, I can understand why people in the trauma business would have hard feelings against a cop killer. Like EMTs and other first responders, cops are part of the trauma community. That's especially true in big-city trauma centers. When I was at Washington Hospital Center, no less than 40 percent of our trauma patients were victims of gunshot or knife wounds; at County-USC in LA it was 25 percent. (In Tucson, by comparison, it's about 13 percent.) And since almost every shooting or stabbing involves a crime, cops are a fixture at the trauma center.

Sometimes they're there to guard a victim or to try to get information about who shot or stabbed them; sometimes they're there to keep an eye on a bad guy who committed a crime and then somehow wound up on the wrong end of a gun or a knife. I've often had cops wearing surgical caps and gowns standing in the OR watching while I'm trying to patch up some accused murderer, even though the guy is under anesthesia and definitely isn't going anywhere. It wasn't at all unusual for me to make the rounds of the surgical ICU and find one of my patients handcuffed to the bed, with a cop standing by to keep an eye on him until he was well enough to be transferred to a medical jail facility.

I like cops in general, and I have to thank them for doing what is often a thankless job. Sure, once in a while you'll encounter a problem officer. For example, the EMTs might bring in some guy who is bleeding and dying and handcuffed to the gurney, and we need to have the cuffs taken off so we can treat him and save his life, but the cop will take his time about it, acting like he's having a hard time finding his cuff key or whatever. That pisses us off. A cop who does that isn't doing his job—just like the backup surgeon I mentioned previously wasn't doing his job.

But most of the time, cops and trauma center staffers get along pretty well. We're all part of that netherworld of violence and blood that most people never see except on TV dramas, so there's a sense of shared experience. There's also the knowledge on the cops' part that if they get shot in the line of duty, we're going to be the ones trying to save their lives.

Recently in Tucson we had a police sergeant who was shot in the head while responding to a burglar alarm call in the early-morning hours. He was just standing there when a bullet came out of the darkness and hit him in the brain. We managed to save him, and four weeks later he was discharged to begin rehabilitation. Medically it was very similar to the Gabby Giffords case, and another example of how far we've come in treating traumatic brain injuries. The police officer is now walking, talking, smiling, and eager to get back on the job.

But such cases don't always turn out so well. I had another case where a cop was shot in the eye with an assault rifle during a crosstown shooting spree by a paranoid schizophrenic dressed in military-style cammies—yet another case of a nut with a gun. The bullet pierced the officer's brain. We managed to keep him alive just long enough for his family members to say good-bye. In a way it was like losing one of our own.

Cops and trauma surgeons—most of them, anyway—also share the sort of rough, twisted sense of humor that helps you deal emotionally with never-ending human tragedy. I remember coming into the trauma bay one time and seeing half a dozen cops gathered around a guy who'd gotten in a wild shoot-out with them, with the cops firing dozens of rounds, and when I examined him I found that he had been shot twenty-four times in his arms and legs. The cops hit everything except his head and torso.

"Not one in the ten-ring," I told the cops. "You guys need more time on the range." They all got a big laugh out of that one.

Of course, it may not sound all that funny here—and there are a million other examples of trauma bay gallows humor that would sound even less so. The idea of a trauma surgeon cracking jokes in the midst of carnage and human suffering bothers a lot of people. Maybe it's okay to do it on a TV doctor show, and they'll laugh right along with it, but not in real life.

But real life is exactly when you have to laugh, even if it's about the terrible things people do to themselves and others. (The exception is with little kids. No one ever jokes about the little kids.) As the old saying goes, if you don't laugh, you'll cry— and as a trauma surgeon, sometimes I would want to cry at the sheer volume of violent injuries that came through the doors every day. And it's especially frustrating when you start seeing the same players coming through the doors over and over again.

I remember one guy, twenty years old, who was brought into Washington Hospital Center with a knife sticking out of his belly, a bayonet-style knife with a blade about ten inches long, the tip of which was embedded in his spine. According to the cops he was a slinger, a small-time drug dealer, who had made the mistake of trying to set up shop on someone else's corner. Usually guys who did that were shot, but in this case one of his competitors stuck a blade in him.

He was definitely going to need a laparotomy, a procedure in which you cut the belly wide open and go in to examine and repair the damage to intestines, liver, kidneys, and other organs. But when the nurses cut his clothes away and I saw the guy's belly, I groaned. The knife was sticking up out of the zipperlike band of thick scar tissue left over from his last laparotomy, which he'd gotten as a result of a gunshot wound the year before. He also had old scar tissue from a bullet wound in the shoulder and another, earlier bullet wound in the hip. This was the guy's fourth visit to the Washington Hospital Center trauma center in the past three years.

There are two problems associated with operating on a guy with a knife sticking out of his latest lap zipper. One is that scar tissue is tough to cut through and even tougher to close. True, the scarring adhesions from the patient's last brush with violent death can reduce the internal bleeding, but cutting your way in there to fix the problem is difficult. The other problem is that even while you're working so hard to fix him, you know there's a good chance you'll have to work on him again sooner or later—or else you'll be working on the guy that he goes out and shoots or stabs in retaliation for sticking the knife in him in the first place.

But that's the way it is in big-city trauma: today's victim is often tomorrow's perpetrator, and vice versa. It starts to seem like the doors to the trauma center aren't swinging but revolving. And virgin chests and bellies, those with nice, clean, unscarred skin, start to seem like the exception and not the rule in some places. You still do the best you can, but it gets a little frustrating when people apparently fail to learn anything from painful experience—extremely painful experience.

Frustrating, too, are the trauma patients who are in serious need of help but fight you when you try to give it to them. A surprising number of patients—surprising to anyone who hasn't worked in a trauma center, anyway—will violently resist any attempt to treat them, even as they're bleeding onto the floor. They'll spit, kick, curse, scream, do anything they can to make your job difficult. Often it's because of drugs or alcohol, but sometimes it's just because they're assholes. Usually the nurses and attendants can eventually get them calmed down with soft words and sedatives, but not always.

I remember one guy, another street player, a huge young guy, who came in bleeding from a superficial gunshot wound to the arm and the left side of his abdomen, near his hip. He had arrived by "homeboy ambulance"—that is, his friends had piled him into a car, brought him in, and then took off. The guy was barely through the doors when he started screaming to see the mother-effing doctor right effing NOW! And when the nurses explained that I'd be there in a minute, he went berserk—mother-effer this and mother-effer that and "I'm going to eff you up!" And on and on. He was scaring the hell out of the nurses and the techs. We finally got him calmed down and he started to let us treat him. But when my X-ray tech went near his head, he grabbed him and started making more threats.

That pushed a button with me that day; I had had enough. I had already assessed him and knew that the gunshot wound to his side hadn't hit anything of concern, that it was going to be just a flesh wound. So I grabbed a couple of beefy hospital security guys and went in and told the guy if he didn't shut up and cooperate I was going to throw him out of my trauma bay. I guess he didn't believe me, because his response was "Eff you!" So the security guys grabbed him and under my direction took him, still bleeding, to the trauma bay doors and pushed him out like some old Western sheriff throwing a drunk through the swinging doors of a saloon. Naturally, as soon as he was out the door, while I stood there waving bye-bye, the guy turned around and started screaming that he was going to sue me.

Of course, even though I knew the guy wasn't going to bleed to death, physically hurling a bleeding patient out the trauma center doors is not considered standard accepted medical practice. The nurses could hardly believe it, but I didn't care. Maybe it was my military background, but nobody threatens my troops.

Sometimes trauma patients will seem to be fighting you when in fact they're simply panicked and struggling to escape the terrible situation they're in; they just want to get away. The adrenaline kicks in, and they are just fighting for their lives. And sometimes they fight because they think you're trying to kill them.

One particular case stands out in my memory. It was a young guy, eighteen years old, who had made the mistake of selling fake heroin to the wrong people. The angry buyers got a sawed-off shotgun, put the guy on his knees, put the shotgun six inches from his face, pulled the trigger, and ran away. It should have been a morgue case, not a trauma center case, but at the last instant the guy had turned his head and the shotgun blast had ripped away his tongue, his teeth, his nose, his cheeks, his eyes. He was still alive because the blast hadn't damaged his brain or his spine; it had simply erased his face.

I'd seen a lot of shockers as a trauma surgeon, but this was one of those "Whoa!" moments. It took me a second or two to process the fact that this guy with no face was still alive. But he clearly was, because he was kicking and struggling with the nurses and attendants who were trying to hold him down flat on his back on the trauma bay gurney.

This was one of the areas where I spent years battling the accepted practices of the civilian and military medical establishment. Standard operating procedure for patients with traumatic injuries to the neck area was for EMTs or medics to strap them down prone on a backboard to immobilize them and prevent damage to the spine. That's fine for a car accident, but when someone is shot in the neck or mouth, what happens? They bleed. And when they're flat on their backs, where does that blood go? It goes down the airway. So when someone is holding them down, they feel like they're drowning, like they're being waterboarded, with their own blood as the water. So they struggle and fight like hell to make it stop.

The solution is simple in cases like that. You forget the backboard and let them sit up, which helps keep the blood from collecting at the back of the throat and going down the airway. I say it's simple, and in practice it is, but what's not simple is getting the medical community—EMTs, nurses, doctors, everybody—to change the way they do things. Sometimes the medical community does things simply because that's the way they've always done them.

In any event, that was what was happening to the young guy with no face; he felt like he was being held down and drowned. I told the nurses to let him sit up, which eased the drowning sensation. Then I took a sucker tube and put it in his hand and guided it to what was left of the back of his mouth so he could clear the blood. He calmed down immediately. We quickly took him up to the OR, still sitting up on the gurney, where we did a tracheostomy under local anesthesia while he was still awake. After we put him under I stopped the bleeding and rearranged what was left of his face with a few sutures to hold it in place until the plastic surgeons could come in and start the reconstruction process.

The case passed out of my hands at that point, so I don't know what happened when the young man finally realized that he was permanently blind and had a face that even after years of plastic surgery would still frighten small children. But that young man had shown a tremendous will to live.

Most trauma patients do the same. Through all the fear and pain, they will fight to live, struggle to hold on to that spark of life. It's when they don't that you know you have a problem.

Whenever I have patients who come in conscious, I try to reassure them. "We're going to take care of you," I'll say. "You're going to be fine." Sometimes the "you're going to be fine" part is the truth and sometimes it's not. Even if they live, if it's obvious they're going to be paralyzed or blind or disfigured or otherwise permanently handicapped, then they're not really going to be "fine." But they want to believe it. It gives them hope and strengthens their will to live.

But sometimes a patient in a trauma bay or ICU room will tell me, "I'm going to die." I don't mean wounded people hysterically screaming, "I'm gonna die! I'm gonna die!"—that happens all the time. I mean patients who look at you and calmly announce, "I think I'm going to die." I hate hearing that, because when patients say they're going to die, it may mean that they are giving up, that they have lost their will to live, or they have a premonition. And more often than not, in a few hours or a few days they'll be dead. It's happened at least a dozen times in my career. There's no scientific basis for it, no correlative studies. But ask any trauma surgeon. When they have that premonition of death, there's a good chance it will come true.

There's another significant cohort of trauma patients who demonstrably have neither the will nor even the desire to live— that is, the attempted suicides. In an average year in America there are about thirty-eight thousand deaths by suicide—nineteen thousand of them by gunshot, nine thousand by hanging or other forms of strangulation, seven thousand by pills or other poisoning, the rest by other means. At the same time, about half a million people a year are admitted to hospital emergency departments for self-inflicted nonfatal injuries, including attempted suicides. Those are the ones we get.

Some people think that an attempted suicide is by definition bogus, that the person didn't really want to kill himself. If he did, they think, he would have done a better job. And we do see a lot of "cutters" with little nicks on the wrist that can be treated with a Band-Aid; sometimes we'll see the same cutter a dozen times in a year. In cases like that, the people don't really want to die. They want attention, and sympathy.

But when a guy puts a gun to his head and pulls the trigger, or cuts an inch-deep gash in his throat or jumps out of a sixth-story window, he's serious. If he survives to be brought to the trauma surgeon, it's only the luck of the draw.

Some might argue that it's a waste of time to treat people like that. If they want to die so badly, why not let them? And besides, they'll probably kill themselves eventually anyway.

But that's actually not true. I've handled hundreds of attempted suicides, and in my experience the majority of people who seriously try to kill themselves are not suffering from chronic mental illness. Instead they're suffering from temporary situational depression—my girlfriend left me, I lost my job, I'm broke—things that time and treatment can heal. Also, the more seriously they hurt themselves, the greater the injury they suffered, the less likely they are to make another attempt—maybe because it hurt so bad the first time. I remember one guy who tried to cut his throat with a circular saw. We managed to save him, but his recovery was incredibly painful—and as far as I know he never tried it again.

There's another category of self-inflicted nonfatal injuries that we often see in the trauma center. Those are the self-mutilators—and that's where it really starts to get weird.

Every trauma surgeon and emergency room physician has seen them: women who jam pencils or scissors or other household items in their vaginas, men who do the same in their rectums, people who intentionally swallow nails or screws, men who put hatpins through their penises or women who try to cut off their nipples. I guess it's a form of Munchausen syndrome, a recognized psychiatric disorder that drives people to feign illnesses and seek out unnecessary surgeries. (We see a lot of those, too: people who will come in complaining of terrible stomach pain or some other problem and demanding that we operate immediately.)

Obviously, people who do those kinds of things need psychiatric help—although sometimes there's a method to their madness. We get a lot of jail inmates who swallow batteries or plastic forks or toothbrushes or otherwise do violence to themselves. I remember one inmate who had more than two dozen abdominal surgeries to remove stuff he had swallowed. The pain from all that surgery must have been horrible, but no one could stop him—and meanwhile, the taxpayers had to pick up the bills. Guys like that are bona fide psych cases, but sometimes you get guys who decide it's easier to do time in a hospital facility than in the jail general population—and safer, too.

I remember one jail inmate, a Hispanic guy, who showed up handcuffed to a gurney with two corrections officers guarding him. It seems the white supremacist Aryan Brotherhood prison gang had put a contract out on him, so to get away he told the jail guards he had swallowed a razor blade. And, sure enough, when they X-rayed him in the jail medical ward there it was, a nice, bright shiny razor blade in his gut. The jail medical staff can handle the small stuff, but when surgery is required they send the inmates to us. When we opened him we found that the guy had hedged his bet a little bit by wrapping tape on the edge of the blade. But still, it had been a pretty desperate move.

He spent a day in the ICU and then they took him back to the prison infirmary.

Anyway, in most serious self-mutilation cases we'll usually put a "psych hold" on them, meaning they can be confined for psychiatric evaluation for up to seventy-two hours. But to confine people for long-term psychiatric treatment against their will is hard to do in our free society. And even if you get a court order for mandatory confinement and treatment, where are you going to treat them? There's a serious shortage of public mental health facilities in this country, so the pressure on administrators to put mentally ill people back on the street is tremendous. That's one reason we have so many chronically mentally ill homeless people wandering the streets. Frankly, I think we as a nation need to be compassionate enough to figure out a better way to force people with serious mental illnesses to get treatment, and be generous enough to pay for it.

Now, so far I've talked about the traumatic injuries that people inflict on themselves or others—gunshots and stabbings. But in fact it's the accidental injuries that really keep the doors of any trauma center swinging.

Car accidents are the worst offenders. As mentioned earlier, every year about thirty-three thousand people in America are killed in motor vehicle accidents, and another 2.5 million are injured. True, we've made some improvements over the years. Seat belts, air bags, and more safety-conscious engineering have helped reduce the number of people killed in car accidents by about 40 percent over the past forty years, even as our overall population has increased. Still, you can't put 250 million passenger vehicles on America's roads and not expect them to regularly run into each other.

For a trauma surgeon, car accidents are actually more medically challenging than shootings or stabbings. With a knife or gunshot wound at least you know where to start. Civilian hand-gun injuries are predictable; the holes usually line up so you can estimate the track of the bullet. True, sometimes a bullet can take a turn if it hits a bone, and once in a rare while you can get bullets that go into the blood vessels and travel. Even more rarely, if you are shot just under the skin from the side and not directly at you, the bullet can sling around and land somewhere unexpected. But usually with a bullet wound you know immediately what you're dealing with.

With a car accident victim it's not so easy. The external injuries may be obvious—a crushed or severed leg, a broken arm—but the potential internal injuries are not. There could be none, or every major internal organ could be damaged. Fortunately, we now have technologies like CT scans and sonograms to give us a look inside you without necessarily having to cut you open. But if you're in a serious crash, there's a good chance you're going to suffer internal damage.

There are a lot of complicated physics principles associated with car crashes, but the simplest way to look at it is that when you're in a car that hits something, the car immediately begins to slow down—but you don't. If you plow head-on into a con-crete wall at sixty miles per hour, your front bumper immediately decelerates to zero, but you're still going sixty miles per hour. Modern cars are designed to dissipate the tremendous energy released in the crash, and seat belts are designed to gradually slow you down. But if you're not wearing a seat belt, you're going to hit the steering column or the dashboard at sixty miles per hour; even if you are wearing a seat belt, at high speed it may not slow you down gradually enough. In either case, the result is that when your body decelerates to zero miles per hour, your movable internal organs—brain, heart, liver, spleen, intestines—are still moving and can suffer extensive damage when they make impact with their supporting structures—skull, sternum, ribs, pelvis. Meanwhile, any loose objects that are in the backseat—a six-pack of Coke, a briefcase, a set of golf clubs—also fly forward at sixty miles per hour, hitting whatever gets in their way, potentially including you, with hundreds or even thousands of pounds of force. And obviously, the greater the speed, the greater the crash forces involved.

Vehicle crashes are also the number-one cause of mass-casualty situations. In fact, when we train for mass casualties, the most common scenario is for freeway pileups, not mass shootings. They can happen anywhere, but they're a particular problem in areas that are prone to heavy fog—or, in Tucson, dust storms. There's a stretch of Interstate 10 outside the city that routinely gets hit with sudden, blinding, zero-visibility dust storms. When a car drives into one at seventy-five miles per hour—that's the legal freeway speed limit in wide-open Arizona—the driver suddenly slams on the brakes, and the guy behind him rear-ends him, then the guy behind him rear-ends him. We had one a while back that involved sixteen wrecked cars and a dozen injured, three of them critically. But our team had trained for just that kind of incident, and all of the injured survived.

But whether it's a single vehicle or a dozen, strange things can happen in car accidents. One of the most puzzling for me involved a man who was killed by an object no bigger than a pencil point.

The patient was a young Navy enlisted man in Seattle who had rolled over his car while on a weekend pass. He hadn't been wearing a seat belt, which is always a bad idea, and he was thrown out the driver's-side window. That should have killed him; people who are thrown from vehicles in a crash are twenty-five times more likely to die than those who are seat-belted in. In fact, his girlfriend was with him in the car and she hadn't been wearing a seat belt either; she died at the scene. But miraculously, the young sailor wasn't badly hurt, just bruised and scuffed up all over.

At the trauma center we did X-rays and CT scans and all the other tests on him, and everything looked fine. When I took over his care, he was naturally distraught over the death of his girlfriend, but his only physical complaint was that he couldn't move his shoulder very well—which was not unusual after a car accident. In fact, I was a little surprised that the residents had even admitted him to the hospital. Since he was in the Navy, they were making arrangements for him to be transferred to the Naval Hospital in Bremerton, and I was planning to discharge him the next day. But as I was driving in to work, I got a call from the senior resident: "Dr. Rhee, your patient is dying."

Dying? From scrapes and bruises? I couldn't believe it. But it was true. It turned out that when he hit the ground after being thrown from the car, a tiny, eighth-inch-long sliver of wood that was lying on the ground had been driven under the skin in his shoulder. It didn't show up on any of the scans, and you couldn't see any exterior sign of it because of the contusions. But the splinter had infected the tissue and the young man had gone into toxic septic shock, and although we operated multiple times over the next two days and pumped in antibiotics, we couldn't stop the rare flesh-eating infection that had developed. The young man died. Here he had somehow survived intact a crash that had left his car a pile of twisted, jagged metal, and he was killed by a tiny speck of wood. That one shook me.

As you might expect, one of the worst kinds of vehicle accidents are car-versus-motorcycle crashes—and the motorcycle almost always loses. Cars making left-hand turns and not seeing the motorcycle bearing down on them are the most common occurrences. Those injuries are especially bad because the motorcycle rider hits the turning car head-on and his pelvis goes flying into the handlebars. That's bad for many reasons, but the worst part is that pelvic fractures can often leave a male rider impotent for the rest of his life. It makes me glad that I sold my BMW 1300c when I left LA. As far as I'm concerned, a trauma surgeon on a motorcycle is like a heart surgeon smoking.

But as bad as vehicle crashes are, vehicle-versus-pedestrian collisions are even worse. Every year about four thousand pedestrians in the US are killed and seventy thousand injured by being hit by cars. The physics involved in a four-thousand-pound car going forty miles per hour and hitting a 180-pound man are painfully obvious. Almost always the pedestrian will have broken legs and pelvic fractures, and if his head hits the windshield of the car, there's a good chance he's going to die. And although it's an unequal contest, sometimes a driver who hits a pedestrian can be hurt as well. I had one case where a car hit a pedestrian and he flew up and crashed headfirst through the windshield, and then the driver was injured when she flew forward and hit her head against the pedestrian's head. She survived; the pedestrian didn't.

Most vehicle injuries and fatalities in the US are preventable—that is, they wouldn't have happened if people weren't driving drunk or driving too fast. About ten thousand people are killed in the US every year in alcohol-related vehicle crashes, another ten thousand in speed-related crashes. Many of those victims are innocent, nondrinking, nonspeeding drivers or passengers who are just in the wrong place at the wrong time and wind up paying for someone else's bad behavior.

But sometimes accidents just happen. I had a good friend, a retired trauma surgeon in Phoenix who had also served in the Navy, who had helped me set up the trauma program in Tucson. He'd been reluctant to do it—he was enjoying his retirement—but we were desperate; in those early days we just didn't have enough trauma surgeons to go around. So finally he agreed, and he started commuting between Phoenix and Tucson for a few days' work in the trauma center each week. Funny thing was, pretty soon he started really getting into it, working more and more and being retired less and less. I guess it's like the firehouse-dog syndrome: a trauma surgeon never loses the sense of excitement when the alarm goes off.

In any event, he was rejuvenated by being back in the trauma fray, and was even working on a research grant to study the use of stem cells in traumatic spinal cord injuries. Then one day he was driving from Phoenix to Tucson and had some irregular heartbeats and he passed out and his car crashed into an embankment, breaking his neck and leaving him paralyzed. It was a hard blow to everyone who knew him, and a terrible irony. Here he was, a trauma surgeon who had spent much of his life treating people with spinal cord injuries, who was trying to find new ways to help them, and then suddenly, out of the blue, through no fault of his own, he was one of them.

It's that random quality, the fact that they can happen anytime, anywhere, to anyone, that makes car accidents so scary.

Of course, cars and motorcycles aren't the only source of painful or deadly accidents. So are ladders, electric appliances, lawn mowers—almost anything can be dangerous if you don't watch what you're doing. I had one guy who was working on a table saw in his garage and his shirt got caught in the blade, pulling him directly onto the saw and ripping his belly open. He came in with a big white dressing on his belly that the EMTs had put there, and when I took that off I could see his entire abdominal cavity, with the intestines ripped completely apart. That was a long and difficult case.

Sometimes accidents take on a kind of regional flair. For example, in Seattle we seemed to get a lot of commercial fishermen who got their hands caught in winches, or impaled themselves with hooks, or fell overboard and got sucked into the boat propeller. In LA we got a lot of Jet Skiers and surfers who crashed into rocks or pier pilings.

Southern Arizona especially produces some odd injuries, things you don't see in most other urban trauma centers. For example, all-terrain-vehicle injuries are an almost daily occurrence, including too many involving kids. People will put their kids on the back of those things and think that just because they're wearing a helmet, they're safe—which they aren't. Again and again I've had kids come in with a pancreas or a liver split in two from a low-speed ATV rollover, only to have the parents say, "I had no idea it was so dangerous." Sometimes the local flora can also play a dangerous role. I had one guy who was thrown off an ATV and was impaled on a cholla cactus, which has spines that can pierce you like stilettos. The paramedic rescue team had to cut the cactus down and air-evac the guy to us with the cactus plant still stuck to him.

Horse-related injuries are a big thing in Arizona as well. A rodeo rider will get his fingers torn almost completely off if he gets them caught between the rope and the saddle horn while he's roping a steer. A bucking bronc rider will come down wrong and get a saddle horn up his rectum. A thousand-pound horse will take a spill on a trail ride and roll over the rider, with predictably disastrous results. It's not the sort of thing we had to worry about much in LA or Washington, DC.

Well, I could go on, but I think you get the point. Coming through those trauma center doors is an endless parade of pain and anguish and suffering. And yet, when I think about it, it sometimes seems like the worst suffering takes place not in the trauma bays but in the waiting room.

Hardly anybody is completely alone in the world. With some exceptions, almost everybody has someone who cares about him—a spouse or girlfriend, a parent or grandparent, a brother or cousin, or maybe just a friend. And when the person they care about is seriously injured, they rush to the hospital—sometimes in ones or twos, sometimes in entire extended families. There's nothing they can really do when they get there. We can't let them into the trauma bays, where they would get in the way or maybe get completely hysterical. All they can do is sit in the waiting room and wait for someone to tell them something. A hospital administrator will get information about the patient from them, and a charge nurse may be able to tell them if their loved one is in the operating room or is on the way to the ICU. But they can't give them details about a trauma patient's medical condition.

That's my job. As the trauma surgeon, after I'm finished treating the patient it's up to me to give the family members the good news, or the sort-of-good news, or the worst news. The family members expect it. They want to hear it from the doctor.

The good news is easy. I'll take them into a separate room, and after making sure I've got the right people, I'll tell them that their son/daughter/spouse/parent/friend is going to be fine. I'll explain in general terms what happened to them, and what we did to treat them, and how we'll manage the recovery. The reactions run the gamut. Sometimes people will cry with relief, sometimes they'll laugh with the release of nervous tension. Often the women will hug me and the men will grab my hand and keep shaking it and shaking it like they can't let go, thanking me all the while. The one question they always ask is: when can we see him?

The sort-of-good news—the news that their injured loved one is alive, but has suffered what may still be a life-threatening or life-changing injury—is more difficult. I try to be as optimistic as possible—it serves no purpose not to be—but often it's still too early for me to know which way it's going to go. Traumatic brain-injury cases are especially difficult. I may suspect that the patient is going to be in a permanent vegetative state, but if I say that, there always seems to be at least one family member who'll say something like, "Dad wouldn't want to live that way," and then demand that we immediately pull the plug, even though it's way too early for that decision. Sadly, the family members who get the sort-of-good news are left in a kind of emotional limbo. They're happy that their loved one is still alive—but for them the waiting is just beginning.

But for the family members to whom I have to give the worst news, the waiting and the hoping are over. I have to tell them that their son/daughter/spouse/parent/friend is dead.

Dead. Under the protocols, I have to use the word. I can't use euphemisms, I can't say things like "We've lost him" or "He's passed on." If I do, they may say, "Well, go find him," or "Who'd you pass him on to?" If they're given any small opportunity for denial, any ray of hope, they'll grab for it, and it just makes it worse. So I have to be clear, concise, final—and no word in the English language has quite the finality of the word *dead*.

Again, the reactions vary. Some people scream, some collapse, some remain so stolid and impassive that I wonder if they actually heard me. Sometimes they get angry. I had one extended family, maybe twenty people, all relatives of a young man shot down in a gang fight, go absolutely berserk, tearing up the waiting room, kicking over tables, smashing the wall-mounted TV. I've never been physically attacked after telling someone that their loved one was dead, but sometimes people will scream and shout curses at me. But they aren't really angry at me. They're angry at the world, at fate, and I just happen to be the one standing there.

But whatever the reaction, I hate doing it. I've had to do it a thousand times, and I still hate it. I hate it when a patient dies, and I hate having to tell someone who cared about him that he's dead. No matter how badly the person was injured when he got to me, no matter how medically hopeless the case, it always feels like failure.

There are other things to hate about being a trauma surgeon. One is dealing with the nonmedical factors that have engulfed the medical profession in recent decades—insurance companies, regulators, administrators, tort lawyers, all looking over your shoulder. Hand in hand with that is the mountain of paperwork—or, now, computer work—that comes with every patient. It seems like we spend about 50 percent of our time trying to save injured people's lives, and the other 50 percent documenting how we did it.

And of course the hours are brutal, especially when like me you're an academician and a research scientist as well as a practicing trauma surgeon. For example, in Tucson I'm not only on call as a working surgeon in the trauma center for thirty-six hours at a stretch, but I also have "day jobs" as the University Medical Center Trauma Medical Director, Professor of Surgery, Vice Chair of Clinical Affairs for the Department of Surgery, Surgical Critical Care Director, Surgical Critical Care Fellowship Program Director, and Pediatric Intensive Care Unit Surgical Co-Director. It doesn't leave a lot of time for family, much less golf.

But I knew all that coming into the job. And the truth is that even after all these years, and all those thousands of patients, every time my phone goes off and I get a text message about another trauma coming in, I still feel the same sense of exhilaration, the same sense of being desperately needed, that I felt when I was a young surgical resident pulling my first trauma shift.

After all my years as a trauma surgeon, sometimes I feel like I'm getting old.

But the job never does.

CHAPTER 6

WAR

Like everyone else in America that morning, on September 11, 2001, I watched transfixed as the second plane flew into the World Trade Center in New York on live television. Also like everyone else, I sensed that life in America would never be quite the same.

But unlike most other Americans, I knew that as an active duty military man, I would be going back out on deployment.

I had just gotten home the night before, September 10, after spending the previous six months at sea as part of the medical team aboard the USS *Boxer*, an amphibious assault ship that served as a floating base of operations for a Marine Expeditionary Unit (MEU). When combined with Navy ships, it forms an "Amphibious Task Force" comprising some 2,200 Marines and 2,500 sailors. Amphibious task forces are America's 911 teams, the first responders, designed to quickly deploy to any hot spot in the world and put American military power on the sea, in the air, and on the ground if necessary.

It had been quite a voyage. The *Boxer* and its accompanying ships had steamed some forty-five thousand miles in the Western Pacific and the Persian Gulf, with training and liberty stops in Australia, Singapore, Thailand, Kuwait, and other ports. Again, it was peacetime, so my medical role as a surgeon wasn't particularly onerous. The bars in Phuket, Thailand, posed a greater threat to the health and safety of our sailors and Marines than any foreign enemy did—or so we thought at the time. In fact, our most intense medical mission was a humanitarian one—that is, providing aid to the embattled nation of East Timor.

East Timor was a breakaway region of Indonesia that had for years been wracked by civil war. In 1999 the Australians had intervened militarily to stop the violence, and later the United Nations and the United States had maintained ongoing operations to provide humanitarian and medical aid—which is where the *Boxer*'s Navy medical staff came in. Every day my medical team and I would ride in from the ship on the gigantic hovercrafts designed to land Marines and their tanks on the shore, then march in formation to the ground transport site where trucks and vans would pick us up and take us to clinics to work.

But frankly, it was a losing proposition. East Timor was incredibly hot, incredibly humid, incredibly dirty, and it boasted the thickest swarms of mosquitoes I had ever seen; it was a miserable place to work. The local health system had completely collapsed, with most of the hospitals destroyed in the fighting and almost all of the local doctors sent fleeing for their lives; there were exactly three Timorese doctors in the entire country of 780,000 people when we got there. The only health care workers were UN and World Health Organization doctors. Some surgical procedures were done, but mostly we delivered supplies to local clinics, everything from rubber gloves to antibiotics to a bathroom scale for weighing pregnant moms to track their progress.

The enormity of the health challenge was frustrating. Really, the people there didn't need toothbrushes and surgical gloves: they needed electricity and roads and clean water, all of which were beyond our abilities to provide. Our Navy medical teams treated more than a thousand people while we were there, for all kinds of illnesses, but mainly for malaria. I guess we did some good, but it was a very small drop in a seemingly bottomless bucket.

Finally we headed for our home base in San Diego, with just a few more stops on the way, including Guam and Hawaii. At Pearl Harbor I got permission from the task force commodore to fly home so I could deliver a long-scheduled scientific talk on our research into suspended animation at the national meeting of the American Association for the Surgery of Trauma. It was a really big deal for me, and I was pretty excited about it. It meant I would miss the big homecoming celebration for the fleet, which was always fun, but the chance to give a presentation at our national meeting made it more than worth it. I would have my own celebration at home.

So I flew into San Diego on September 10, and Emily picked me up and took me home. They had the whole house decorated with homecoming banners and signs: WELCOME HOME, DADDY! I couldn't believe how much Michael and Anna had grown in just six months. I was exhausted, and I wound up passing out pretty early that night. At six A.M. the next morning I was still in bed when Emily came running in and said in a hurried voice, "Turn on the TV!" Seconds after the TV news came on, I saw an airplane crashing into a building in New York.

Our country was at war. And I was eager to get into the fight.

That may be a little hard for people in the civilian world to understand. It's not that you want there to be a war. But if there is a war, as a military man you desperately want to be a part of it. It's what you trained for, what you've been paid to be ready to do throughout your military career. To be stuck on the sidelines while there's a war going on is like being a fireman who never gets to fight a fire.

And to be truthful, I thought they needed me in the fight. After all, I had handled more trauma cases in the past six years than anyone else in Navy medicine—largely because there were hardly any other Navy surgeons who were doing trauma. At that time there were only six board-certified trauma surgeons in the US Navy—that's right, six. So it only seemed logical that the Navy would send me where there were going to be trauma cases. Also, in recent years I had been deeply involved in developing what was known as the Navy Forward Resuscitative Surgical System, which was designed to reduce the time it took to get a wounded Marine to a surgical operating room. Instead of working in hospitals in the rear, the mobile FRSS teams—two surgeons, an anesthesiologist, a nurse, and an OR tech—would move right behind the Marine combat units, setting up and manning OR tents as close to the fighting as possible. I had spent many hours in the field with the Marines, figuring out what equipment the FRSS teams needed, how to pack it, how to move it, how to set it up.

In short, then, if the Navy was going to send a surgeon into the fight, I figured I was the logical guy.

Unfortunately, when it comes to the Navy bureaucracy, logic often fails to win the day. My post–USS *Boxer* assignment was as an attending surgeon and head of Surgical Critical Care at the Balboa Navy Hospital in San Diego—and that's where the Navy intended me to stay. As far as they were concerned, I had had my tour of sea duty and now it was the next guy's turn.

Then I caught a break. A couple of months after the New York and Washington attacks, the 15th Marine Expeditionary Unit out of Camp Pendleton, which had replaced my earlier MEU in the Persian Gulf, was ordered to set up a forward operating base at a small former Taliban outpost about seventy miles southwest of Kandahar in Afghanistan. Later named Camp Rhino, it was the first conventional US ground force base in the country. The break for me was that the sole surgeon attached to the MEU at Camp Rhino had to come home for medical reasons. When I heard they needed a replacement surgeon ASAP, I pulled some strings and got the temporary assignment. Emily wasn't as happy about it as I was; I had been home for only about three months and it was time for me to go again. But she understood. I packed up four duffel bags full of gear—cammies, boots, everything I thought I would need, including a folding chair and a compact air mattress. Having been in the field with the Marines during training so many times, I knew how important those small comforts could be. One thing I didn't take was my MOPP (Mission Oriented Protective Posture) gear, the bulky, specially treated suit, gas mask, and rubber galoshes US troops wore as protection against chemical and biological attacks. Biochem attacks were the big fear at that time, but I figured if we got "slimed" with chemicals or biologicals, I would be toast anyway. Besides, if I took the MOPP gear I wouldn't have had room for my air mattress and folding chair.

Anyway, I flew commercial from San Diego to Kuwait, then an Air Force C-130 to Pakistan and on to Rhino, arriving there in December of 2001. There wasn't much to Camp Rhino, just a few warehouses and hangars and administrative buildings surrounded by a ten-foot fence; reportedly it had been used as an opium processing and distribution center before the Americans arrived. Set in the middle of a dry lake bed, beyond the camp perimeter there was nothing but mile after mile of flat, treeless, waterless, uninhabited landscape stretching to the horizon without a sign of life; there weren't even any bugs. It was like being on the surface of the moon.

Camp Rhino wasn't big on amenities, either. Unlike the vast, well-appointed bases the US would later build, there was no chow hall, no MWR (morale, welfare, and recreation) facility, no fast-food outlets, no showers, no laundry facilities. Marines slept on the concrete floors of the warehouses or in "fighting holes"— the Marine term for foxholes—they dug in the dirt. Chow was MREs, Meals Ready to Eat, also known as Meals Refused by Everyone—and, because of their high-starch, low-fiber content, Meals Refusing to Exit. Every drop of water had to be flown in and was for drinking purposes only; bathing was performed with baby wipes, if you had them. They eventually flew in some plywood and made one shitter, a plywood box with four holes cut out over fifty-five-gallon drums cut in half. When the drums were full, they were dragged out and the contents were doused with JP-8 fuel and set afire; the smell hung over the camp like a literal shit mist.

But I couldn't have been happier. At age forty I was like a kid on a camping trip. Just like my time at Pendleton years earlier when I was a medical student, and in other field exercises with the Marines, I got to hang out with a great bunch of guys, and I gained some experience in maintaining a surgical unit in a remote, windswept, dusty outpost. Another nice thing about Camp Rhino was that it was a long way from the flagpole— military-speak for being far removed from headquarters brass— so there wasn't a lot of silly, rear echelon military-regulation stuff, no shining of belt buckles or maintaining a straight gig line. The only things we really had to keep clean were the two medical tents, one of which was the operating room. Given the clouds of dust kicked up by the wind and the helicopters and the tramping of booted feet, this was never easy. We tried to keep our weapons clean by sticking foam earplugs into the muzzles, although the line Marines hated it when we did that.

Despite that, the Marines let us medical guys go out to what we called the range—actually, it was just another patch of barren desert—and shoot as much as we wanted to. Those were the good times. Once I told the MEU operations officer I wanted to take my people out for a little weapons-proficiency practice, and he gave me an ammo box with a thousand rounds of 9-millimeter pistol ammo—which would cost about four hundred bucks at a stateside sporting goods store—and told me that we weren't allowed to bring any of it back. By the time I loaded and fired all those rounds my thumbs were blistered and bleeding from loading our magazines. I also got to shoot a new .50-caliber sniper rifle that some of the Marine sniper guys brought, which was very cool.

But the coolest thing I got to do came when Camp Rhino was being shut down, and I got to go out with the EOD (Explosive Ordnance Disposal) guys and blow up some of the excess mortar rounds and other ordnance the Marines couldn't take with them. (That sounds wasteful, but in fact it would have cost the taxpayers more for the Marines to move the ordnance than to destroy it.) We piled up a defective Hellfire missile and dozens and dozens of mortar rounds in a pit wired with C-4 explosive, and the EOD guys let me, "the doc," pull the fuse cord. It was a three-minute fuse, and after I activated it I started walking toward the EOD Humvee that was supposed to take us out of the blast area—or at least I started out walking. But the more I thought about the five hundred pounds of high explosives at my back, the faster I walked, until finally I broke into a dead run for that Humvee, while the EOD guys inside were laughing their asses off. When that thing went off it sent up a mushroom cloud like a mininuke and cracked every remaining windowpane in Camp Rhino.

Good times.

Medically, my time at Rhino wasn't too demanding. Before I got there, three Marines from the unit who had been operating around Kandahar had been wounded by a mine, with one of them losing a leg. But mostly the Navy medical team treated the usual injuries and illnesses that afflict any group of eleven hundred Marines: broken bones, sprained ankles, lower GI problems. The good news was that by the time we got to Rhino, Al-Qaeda and the Taliban were on the run, knocked out of power by their local Afghan enemies with the critical assistance of US special operations teams. Eventually the Taliban would regroup and start to wage bloody insurgent war against US troops, but while I was at Camp Rhino, from December 2001 to February 2002—another Christmas at home missed—not a single Marine was killed or wounded by hostile fire there. I had expected to gain experience in treating military trauma cases during my deployment, but I certainly wasn't disappointed that I hadn't.

Still, I knew that it wasn't over, that what was being called the global war on terrorism (the GWOT) wasn't finished, that the fight would continue in Afghanistan and possibly elsewhere. I knew there was going to be a continuing need for Navy medical personnel who were experienced in treating trauma. More significantly, the US military finally understood that, too.

After Camp Rhino closed down, I spent a couple of months in Dubai before I finally got back to San Diego, fully expecting to resume my duties as head of critical care at Balboa Hospital. But Rear Admiral James Johnson, head of the Navy medical system in San Diego, had other ideas.

For years I and the other Navy trauma surgeons had been campaigning for a program that would take Navy medical personnel—doctors, nurses, technicians, corpsmen—and temporarily put them to work in civilian trauma centers, just as I had done in Seattle and Washington, DC. The idea was to give them some real-life experience in treating bullet wounds and other traumatic injuries, things that they had never had to handle in the peacetime Navy medical system. It would at least give them an idea of what they might encounter in a combat zone—and after years of peace, they really needed it.

After the first Persian Gulf War, the Pentagon had made some halfhearted efforts to establish such a program, but it never really got off the ground. The logistics were difficult. The money was scarce. Surgeons were scarce. To pull surgeons out of their regular jobs and send them away for a prolonged period of training was expensive, and there was resistance to extended training away from home.

But the global war on terror gave it new urgency. And Admiral Johnson, who was himself a surgeon, had the clout to make it happen. After reviewing and evaluating various civilian trauma centers, the Navy chose LA County–University of Southern California Medical Center—known for short as County-USC—in the Boyle Heights area east of downtown Los Angeles as the site for the new program. (The Army set up a similar program in Miami, and the Air Force in Baltimore.) And Admiral Johnson wanted me to go up there and run it.

I have to admit, I was a bit ambivalent about it. Yes, it was exactly what I and other Navy trauma surgeons had been pushing for, and the prospect of setting up the program and running it was professionally exciting. And I knew how much my experience in civilian trauma centers had benefited me, and how valuable that experience would be if I ever got into the fight. I wanted other Navy personnel to have that same experience.

On the other hand, with all due respect to the good people of LA, Emily and I weren't wild about the idea of abandoning the quiet, peaceful, perfect life on Coronado Island for the smoggy rat race of the LA megalopolis. But in the end I couldn't pass it up—and in fact I really had no choice. I figured if I turned down Admiral Johnson's request, my Navy career would be down the drain. So in July 2002 we moved up to LA and I became director of the Navy Trauma Training Center (NTTC) at County-USC.

The twenty-story, art deco–style County-USC building was built in the 1930s, and over the years the iconic structure has probably become the most photographed hospital in the country. Its exterior was used in TV shows from *Dr. Kildare* to *General Hospital,* and numerous movies and TV shows were shot in and around it. It was what an entire generation of Americans thought a hospital should look like.

But as a functioning hospital building, it was a disaster. It was old, cramped, and run-down and had suffered structural damage in the 1994 Northridge earthquake. (In 2008 the old building would be replaced by a new one built nearby.) One of the most frustrating things about it was that there was only one elevator in the main tower that we could use to transport patients on gurneys, an old-style elevator that actually had a woman sitting on a chair inside who ran it up and down—not exactly an ideal situation when you're trying to rush a bleeding patient from the ER on the first floor to the OR on the fifteenth floor.

Despite all that, as a trauma training center County-USC had one great advantage over other venues: there was never any shortage of patients. Every year about seven thousand trauma patients were wheeled in through the ER doors, an average of about twenty a day, people who had been shot, stabbed, bludgeoned, crushed in car accidents, injured in industrial or household accidents. A lot of the GSW victims were gang members: Bloods and Crips, 18th Street and White Fence, and on and on, all with their own sets and subsets, all seemingly eager to gun each other down; in all, LA County was home to an estimated eighty thousand bona fide gangbangers. But there was also a steady stream of domestic disputes, armed robbery victims, and of course innocent bystanders, as well as law enforcement officers.

Having the Navy Trauma Training Center at County-USC was a good deal for the hospital. Our trauma training team consisted of ten Navy personnel: a director and trauma surgeon (me), an orthopedic surgeon, an anesthesiologist, an emergency medicine physician, an operating room nurse, an ICU nurse, an emergency medicine nurse, a senior medical corpsman, an operating room technician, and a Medical Services Corps administrator to handle the paperwork. Although we were all being paid by the Navy, when we weren't teaching classes we worked right along with the civilian County-USC emergency department staff, helping with whatever cases came through the doors. We figured that the program was providing LA County with about $5 million of free trauma services every year.

They needed the help, because like most urban trauma centers, County-USC was a madhouse. On my very first Friday night I think we had thirty trauma patients, with nine cases in the OR. I'd be in the OR operating on a guy, and while we were knee-deep in him we'd get a call that another trauma red was coming in, so I'd have to run down fifteen flights of stairs—I couldn't wait for that damned elevator—to get the new patient resuscitated and stabilized, then I'd run back up fifteen flights to the OR, then I'd have to run back down to stabilize another guy, and on and on until the shooters finally went to bed at about six A.M. And then it would start right back up the next night. At the end of a shift spent running up and down between the OR and the ER, I would feel like I had spent twenty-four hours in a combination slaughterhouse and gym.

The ancient Greek physician Hippocrates, creator of the Hippocratic oath, once said that "War is the only proper school for a surgeon." What he meant was that only amid the carnage of war could a surgeon gain the experience needed to truly master his craft.

But with all due respect to Hippocrates, he never pulled a weekend shift at County-USC. It may not have been an actual war zone, but it came pretty close—which was why we picked LA County for the Navy Trauma Training Program in the first place. It was kind of ironic that the military was so lacking in trauma experience that it had to go to an inner-city battle zone to learn how to operate in an actual combat zone.

But it was a big win-win for everybody. The hospital got some badly needed—and free—help. And we got to give Navy medical personnel training that on the battlefield would help save lives.

The plan for the NTTC was to take Navy medical personnel—again, doctors, nurses, technicians, corpsmen—who were scheduled to be deployed to combat zones or to the fleet and put them through a nonstop thirty-day training program in trauma care, both individually and as members of the trauma team. Each class had about thirty students. To get them into the right frame of mind, on a class's first night in LA we would simulate a terrorist attack on their barracks, with smoke bombs and gunfire sounds and strobe lights, and we'd "capture" them and prone them out on the grounds with their hands zip-tied. We were trying to impress upon them that this course was combat training, not hospital training. We were the boot camp of military medicine, and if they didn't always like it, they certainly needed it.

There was a lot of classroom work with lectures and body simulators, but most of the training was hands-on. Corpsmen would be sent out to work shifts with civilian paramedics, flight nurses would work with civilian aircraft medevac units, surgeons and nurses and OR techs would work in the trauma bays and operating rooms. The students were on duty all the time, especially the surgeons.

It was an eye-opening experience for most of them, especially the young corpsmen. They had all had medical training after boot camp, learning how to insert IVs, clear airways, even perform some minor field surgery on simulators. But they had never seen the real thing. So on their first night shift in the ER, when the doors would fly open and the paramedics would wheel in some guy with multiple bullet holes in him, spurting blood, his belly or his chest or his skull torn open, a lot of those kids would get a deer-in-the-headlights look. They'd go into a kind of temporary emotional shock that would cause them to freeze, or even start to get woozy and pass out—which is exactly what we didn't want to happen to them the first time they saw a badly wounded Marine on the battlefield.

But as the course went on, and they saw badly injured people and blood on the floor night after night, they got used to it, desensitized. It wasn't like corpsman school and then being in a quiet clinic somewhere doing immunizations, physicals, eye exams, and laboratory jobs and treating bumps and bruises. It was like being in the battle zone, but without the flak gear.

The more experienced nurses and OR techs and senior corpsmen also benefited. As I said, for decades the Navy medical corps had been practicing peacetime medicine, not wartime medicine, so they could spend years working in Navy hospitals without ever handling a serious trauma case. Again and again I had nurses and techs and senior corpsmen come up to me and say, "Captain, I've been in the Navy for twenty-seven years and this is the first time I've ever seen a bullet wound. I've been everywhere with the Marines, but I never saw a gunshot wound till I got to LA." And later I'd get e-mails from them from the field saying, "Thank you for that training. It helped me save lives."

I remember one e-mail I got from Afghanistan, from a female Canadian military surgeon who had managed to pull some strings and get into our program. Being from Canada, which has strict gun-control laws, she had seldom seen a gunshot wound—but in LA she saw plenty. She had learned how to open the chests of gunshot victims, something we had to do all too often in LA, so when she got to Afghanistan and they brought in a Canadian soldier who'd been shot in the heart she knew what to do, and she saved his life. She wrote to us to express her appreciation, and to thank us on that Canadian soldier's behalf.

But not everyone was so appreciative. Strangely enough, the guys who were most resistant to the trauma training program were the guys who I thought needed it the most—the young Navy surgeons.

It was partly an ego thing. I don't want to shock anybody, but surgeons are sometimes known for having well-developed egos. (I've even been accused of that myself—unfairly, of course.) After all their years of surgical training, they think they know it all.

But they don't. Sure, a colorectal or thoracic surgeon may have gone through a two- or three-month trauma rotation during his residency, but ever since then he'd been doing nice, clean, scheduled surgeries in a quiet hospital OR, not meatball surgery in a chaotic ER or emergency operating room where there might be six guys with serious GSWs stacked up and coding at the same time and thirty people outside screaming and yelling. Putting a general surgeon or a colorectal guy into a mass-casualty trauma situation would be like putting me in an OB-GYN ward with twenty mothers about to give birth at the same time. I would remember the basics from med school and residency, but I would surely make mistakes. I didn't want to send a surgeon who was not prepared out to a battlefield to get on-the-job trauma training when a young Marine's or soldier's or sailor's life was on the line. Sometimes I had to set the surgeons straight about how much they didn't know about trauma. The older (smarter) ones always listened. But the young ones were a pain in the ass.

The Navy medical bureaucracy often didn't help. Time after

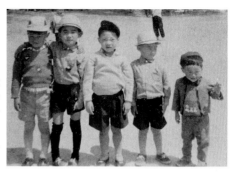

Seoul, South Korea, 1964. That's me, Meong Hoon Rhee, on the right at age three. The name "Peter" would come later. To my right are my cousin Joon Oh; my older brother Hoon Rhee; another cousin, Soon Oh; and an unidentified friend.

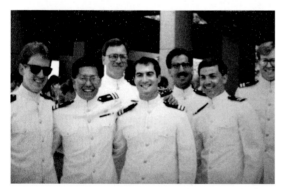

Hospital doctors, nurses, and staff in Tororo, Uganda, in 1969. My father, Dr. Ky Young Rhee, is on the bottom right. My father was a surgeon, which would have a major impact on my life—although I didn't realize it at the time.

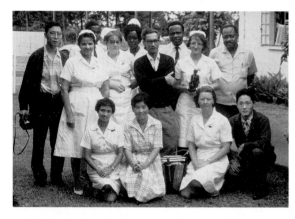

That's me, second from left, with my Navy classmates on graduation day from the Uniformed Services University of the Health Sciences in Bethesda, Maryland, in 1987. One of the reasons we're smiling is that we had all just gotten promoted from ensigns to lieutenants, which meant a nice raise in pay. The commencement was held at the Kennedy Center and the speaker was President Ronald Reagan. He told us, "Yours is the only medical school in America that trains physicians to be ready for duty on the bottom of the ocean or on the surface of the moon and any place in between."

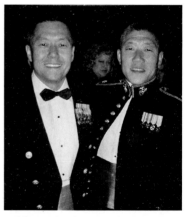

With my brother, Marine Corps Lt. Col. Luke Rhee, at a Marine Corps Birthday Ball in 2001. I had spent a summer with Luke's infantry platoon at Camp Pendleton when I was in medical school and he was a young Marine lieutenant. Even though I was Navy, he made sure his little brother looked and acted like a Marine.

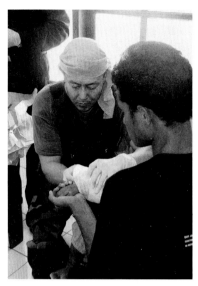

Treating an injured child during a humanitarian mission in East Timor with the crew of the Amphibious Assault Ship USS *Boxer* in 2001. The *Boxer*'s amphibious task force traveled 45,000 miles in the Western Pacific and the Persian Gulf during that deployment. I got back home to San Diego the night of September 10, 2001. The next morning, America was at war.

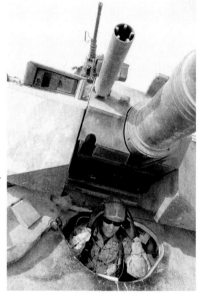

January 2005, at Camp Ramadi, Iraq. This is one of the advantages that military surgeons have over their civilian counterparts. How often does a civilian surgeon get to drive a tank?

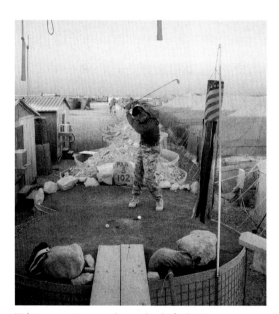

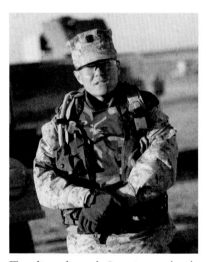

Taking a swing on the makeshift driving range on top of Hesco anti-blast barriers at Camp Taqaddum, Iraq, in October 2005. It was a great stress reliever until a sliced ball hit a general's Humvee and the range was shut down.

Traveling through Iraq in my battle gear in 2005.

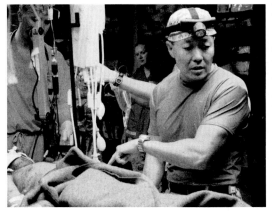

In the OR at "Charlie Med" at Camp Ramadi, Iraq, in 2005. The wounded patient we're treating is an Iraqi enemy insurgent captured by US forces. My firm policy at Charlie Med was that all patients got the best treatment possible, even if they had had the misfortune to be born on the wrong side.

Our Forward Resuscitative Surgical System (FRSS) team at work in the Charlie Med OR at Camp Ramadi in 2005. Our job was to keep the wounded alive and get them stabilized before sending them to the rear for more treatment. Here we're getting a wounded Marine ready to be medevac'ed by helicopter to an Army Combat Support Hospital in Baghdad.

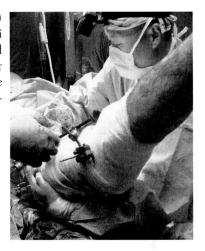

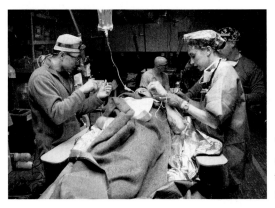

"You're going to be OK." Here I'm explaining his injuries to a postoperative wounded Marine at Charlie Med in January 2005.

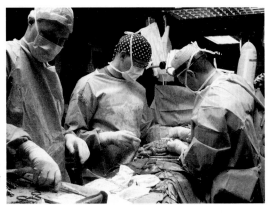

Operating on a wounded American soldier at Charlie Med in December 2005. OR tech Robert Swiatkowski is on the left and Navy surgeon Lt. Cmdr. Cliff Smith is in the center.

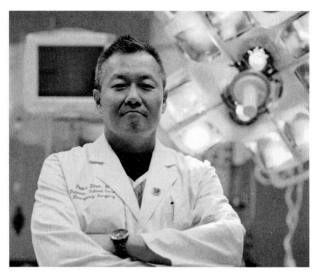

Chief of Trauma at University Medical Center in Tucson, Arizona. Great town, great people—and one of the best trauma teams in America.

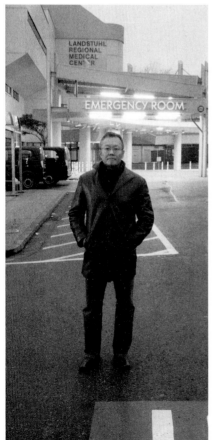

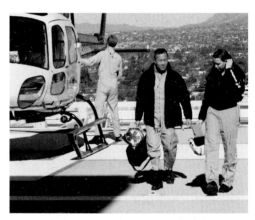

On the helicopter pad on the roof of the UMC Trauma Center after a flight on a LifeNet medical services helicopter. Physician's assistant Sara Peroti and I had been on a tour of the Navajo Nation in Northern Arizona.

Outside the Army's Landstuhl Regional Medical Center in Landstuhl, Germany, in 2010. Many of the US troops wounded in Iraq and Afghanistan came here before going home. Although I was a civilian by then, I still got a chance to serve as a civilian visiting professor and lend the military surgeons a hand.

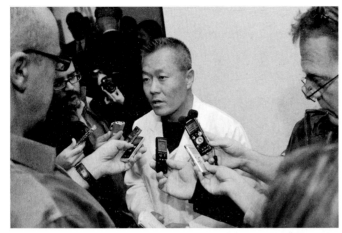

The press descended on University Medical Center after the January 8, 2011, mass shooting. I knew that if I didn't give them as much information as possible they would get their information somewhere else—and it probably would be wrong.

UMC Chief of Neurosurgery Dr. Michael Lemole headed the neurosurgery team that operated on Congresswoman Giffords. Here we are getting ready for another press briefing.

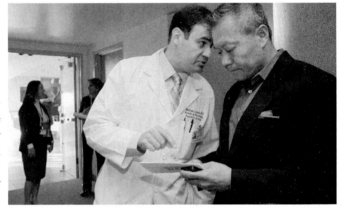

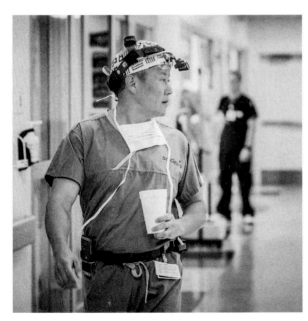

Another day at work at the UMC Trauma Center.

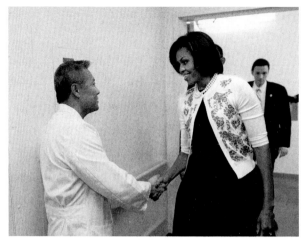

Welcoming First Lady Michelle Obama as she was brought up the back steps of the intensive care unit to visit the patients and staff after the shooting in Tucson.

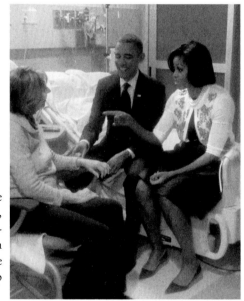

President Obama and Michelle Obama in the ICU talking to gunshot victim Pamela Simon, Congresswoman Giffords's community outreach coordinator. Pam was shot in the arm and left chest. Miraculously, the bullet to the chest missed her vital organs and wound up near her left hip.

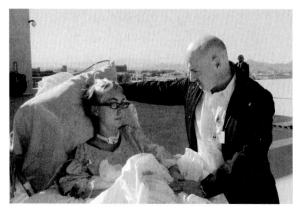

Gabby Giffords and Mark Kelly on the helicopter pad on the roof of the Trauma Center the day before she left for rehabilitation treatment in Houston. Gabby's excursions to the helipad gave her a chance to get some sun and gaze out at the city she loved.

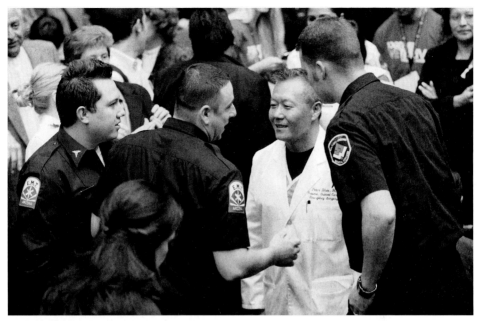

Thanking the first responders at the memorial service for the Tucson shooting victims.

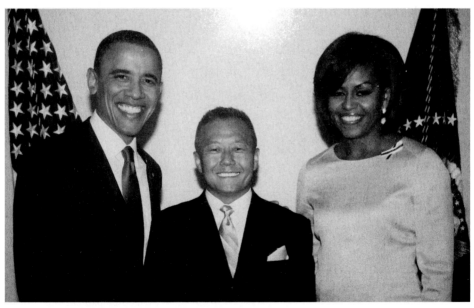

With the president and first lady at the State of the Union Address in 2011. Michelle Obama invited me to sit in her box. They're both really tall.

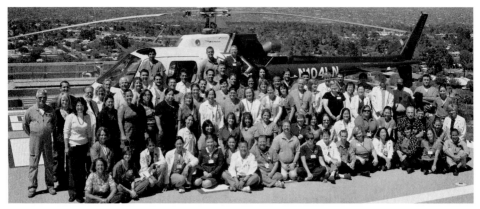

The Tucson trauma team on the trauma center helicopter pad, with me sitting in the middle of the first row. I've never worked with a more dedicated, conscientious, and compassionate group of people.

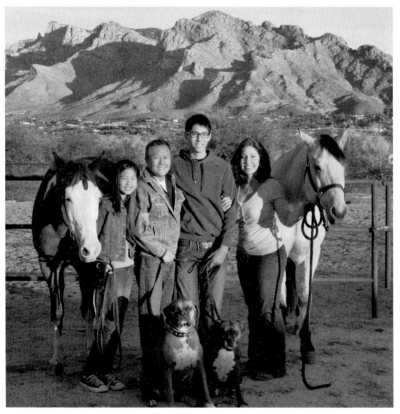

Christmas photo, 2011. My wife calls this "the sixteen eyes" picture. She wanted all of us looking at the camera, which isn't easy when dogs and horses are involved. From left to right are Rose the horse; my daughter, Anna (age eleven); me (age fifty); my son, Michael (age seventeen); my wife, Emily (age unstated); Levi the horse; and in front, the dogs, Kramer and Morgan.

time I'd try to get some surgeon out of a Navy hospital to go through the trauma training, only to have the officer in charge say, "Hey, he's my hernia guy. If I send him to you for a month, who's going to do my hernias?" It was frustrating. I would tell them to find a civilian general surgeon in town and pay him to do the hernias, because the Navy surgeons were needed in the battle zone.

Yes, the trauma training was inconvenient and expensive. But I figured we should let the administrative weenies in the Pentagon worry about that. I was looking at the cost-versus-value of saving the lives of soldiers in the field. The speed and teamwork required in trauma shouldn't be learned on our servicemen in the field during the heat of the battle. People willing to serve our country in war deserve better. I was glad that Admiral Johnson knew what was important, what the priorities were, and backed us all the way.

Still, despite the administrative difficulties, during my time there we ran more than a thousand Navy medical personnel through the trauma training program—and hundreds more would follow. It's hard to quantify, but based on the kind of reports from the field that I mentioned above, I'm convinced that every NTTC graduate who went to the combat zone had learned something that saved lives.

I learned some things, too. Every one of the thousands of trauma patients I handled during my career broadened my breadth of knowledge, helped me understand how to better treat future patients who came through the ER doors. Sometimes the information was cumulative: this worked with patients A, B, and C, so let's try it on patient D. That's why we carefully documented every trauma case and tracked every outcome.

But sometimes we'd stumble onto something that was a dramatic advance in trauma care. One of the best examples of that involved a hemostatic agent (that is, something that stops bleeding) called QuikClot, which was developed by a Connecticut company called Z-Medica, Inc.

QuikClot is a granular powder made from a mineral called zeolite that is known for its absorbent qualities. It looks like kitty litter, and it acts like it, too. When you pour it on a severely bleeding wound, it absorbs the blood fluids and concentrates coagulation factors to make the blood clot up and stop the bleeding. I'd been conducting lab studies to evaluate the use of various hemostatics, and QuikClot had proved to be the most effective in stopping bleeding on external wounds where a tourniquet couldn't be applied. Its primary drawback was that when mixed with a fluid substance like blood, a chemical reaction caused it to heat up, sometimes just a little, sometime enough to burn tissue—although if you're bleeding to death, a little burned tissue is the least of your problems. Based on those studies, in May 2002 we'd gotten the Food and Drug Administration to approve QuikClot within just a few months—usually it takes years—and soon the 3.5-ounce packets of QuikClot were standard-issue throughout the Navy, Marine Corps, and Air Force. (The Army favored another hemostatic compound.)

Anyway, one day early on in the NTTC program I had just finished giving the trainees a lecture on the uses of QuikClot when we got a GSW case. The patient had reportedly attacked some LA cops when they were serving a warrant, and they shot him. Really shot him. He had seven bullet holes in him, and he was bleeding from almost everywhere—chest, belly, everywhere. We got him into the OR on the fifteenth floor; one of the Navy surgeon trainees who'd been in the hemostatics lecture was working on him with me. I had his chest open and his aorta clamped off, we were giving him blood, I was cauterizing, I was sewing up everything I could see, I was packing his chest with sponges.

But I was running out of tricks, his blood pressure was 50 and I couldn't stop the bleeding inside his chest, and he was using up blood that I might have needed to save the next guy who came through the door. Finally I told the anesthesiologist, "Don't give him any more blood, he's a goner. We've got to let him go."

And then the Navy surgeon who was working with me, who had just sat through the hemostatics lecture, said to me, "Why don't you try QuikClot?"

It was like a lightbulb went on over my head. Of course! We'll pour QuikClot into his chest!

True, QuikClot was FDA approved for external use only—it said so in big letters right on the packages—and true, it might cause some tissue burns. But I was about to declare this guy dead, so I had nothing to lose—and more important, he had nothing to lose. I figured that having the guy live and possibly sue me for using a product in an unapproved manner was better than having him not sue me because he was dead.

So I told the anesthesiologist to put a little more blood in him to keep the pressure from dropping any further, and I told the Navy doc to hold pressure on his bleeding by putting two hands inside his open chest and pushing down under his left lung. Meanwhile, I ran off to get some QuikClot. The problem was that the QuikClot was in my office in the NTTC training center on the sixth floor, and we were on the fifteenth floor and there was only that one damn elevator. So I had to run down nine flights of stairs to my office, grab some QuikClot packages, and run back up nine flights to the OR. It took about five minutes, but when I got back the guy was still alive. We poured the QuikClot into his chest and we could feel it getting really hot. But lo and behold, the bleeding stopped, his blood pressure went up, he stabilized. I dove into his abdomen to fix his spleen, kidney, liver, and intestines, and a couple weeks later he walked out of the hospital.

Later we did a study, published in the *Journal of Trauma*, of 103 cases in which QuikClot had been used by military doctors and civilian trauma surgeons and emergency first responders—83 of them involving application to external wounds and twenty cases of internal use by military and civilian surgeons. Overall, QuikClot proved effective in stopping blood loss in 92 percent of the cases, with the other 8 percent involving patients who apparently were already too far gone for the hemostatic agent to do any good. There was some burn scarring in one of the internal-use cases, but again, if you're bleeding to death, that's a small price to pay. Our conclusion was that QuikClot used internally was highly effective.

The point here is that there is always something new to learn about trauma if you're willing to think outside the box and not be tied down to the old ways of doing things just because that's the way they've always been done. That young Navy surgeon who suggested we use QuikClot on that dying man was doing exactly what we were trying to teach in the Navy Trauma Training Program, what you have to do in a fast-paced, chaotic combat situation—improvise, adapt, think on your feet.

It was good training. And, in fact, I'm convinced that the NTTC program came along just in time.

Because just six months after we started the program, America's battle zone suddenly got a whole lot bigger and a whole lot bloodier.

CHAPTER 7

A GOOD BAD DAY
AT CHARLIE MED

The good bad day at Charlie Med started out good enough. The line of plastic Porta-Johns in the company area had just been emptied and hosed out and sprayed with disinfectant, and I was the first one there that morning, which meant I had a nice clean place to relax and ponder the issues of the day.

Believe me, when you're in the combat zone, it's those little things that count.

It was December 7, 2005—Pearl Harbor Day, the anniversary of the Japanese attack on Hawaii—and the end of my first month at Charlie Med, an Echelon II medical facility in Ramadi, Iraq, a dusty city of half a million people situated on the banks of the Euphrates River seventy miles west of Baghdad. Ramadi was both the capital of the vast Anbar Province that covered most of western Iraq and the center of the Sunni anti-US insurgency that was killing and maiming so many young Americans. Charlie Med, short for "C" Medical Company, 228th Forward Support

Battalion of the 2-28th Brigade Combat Team, was a unit of the Pennsylvania Army National Guard charged with providing medical services for US troops fighting in and around the city.

How I wound up there, attached as a Navy surgeon to a Pennsylvania Army National Guard unit, takes a little explaining.

After the invasion of Iraq in March 2003, I was once again champing at the bit to get into the combat zone—and once again the Navy wasn't cooperating. We had started the Navy Trauma Training Center program at County-USC just six months earlier, and it was being widely lauded as a big success. The Navy wanted me to keep on training other surgeons and medical staff in trauma techniques, instead of having me take my trauma skills to the battlefield personally. Professionally, I could understand the argument. Personally, I felt that the combat zone was where I was needed most. I had spent my entire professional life learning how to be a trauma surgeon on the Navy's dime, and now that there was a war on, it was time for me to pay the Navy back. As I said earlier, for me to not be deployed to the war zone was like being a firefighter who wasn't allowed to go near a fire.

Then in the fall of 2005, two and a half years after the war began, I caught a break. The Navy and the II Marine Expeditionary Force, which was then in command of the fight in Anbar Province, found itself short a surgeon and needed a replacement. After pulling a lot of strings and calling in a few favors—I hadn't spent twenty-two years in the Navy for nothing—I got the job. I went down to Camp Pendleton to get my orders cut and draw my gear: cammies, flak vest, Kevlar helmet, and 9-millimeter sidearm.

I was a Navy captain by then, an O–6, the equivalent of a Marine full colonel, which certainly had its privileges.. It usually takes a week to draw combat gear; I got it done in a day. And since I was going in as a replacement surgeon, I got to fly commercial instead of waiting around for military transport. It turned a few heads at the airport when I checked in with four duffel bags full of gear, my weapon (but no ammo) included. But I got on the flight and headed for Kuwait via London. From Camp Victory in Kuwait I got on an Air Force C-130 cargo plane and flew to Al Asad, a sprawling former Iraqi air base a hundred miles west of Baghdad.

By the time I got there, Al Asad had experienced the same rear-area "Americanization" that had taken over other large US bases in Iraq. When American Marines and soldiers first went into Iraq, and earlier Afghanistan, they had lived close to the ground, sleeping in tents or abandoned buildings, eating MREs, crapping in the dirt—roughing it. But at Al Asad there were flush toilets, some showers, a movie theater, gyms, an extensive and well-stocked PX, air-conditioned, prefabricated living quarters called "cans," and fast-food joints ranging from Burger King to KFC to Pizza Hut. Although Al Asad had occasionally taken some fire from mortars or rockets, it was about as far in the rear with the gear as it could be.

(Interestingly, many of the routine security functions at the base were provided by former Ugandan soldiers who worked for a privately contracted security company. When I first encountered some of them and spoke to them in the Swahili phrases I remembered from my youth, they almost fell over in astonishment.)

In short, then, life at Al Asad was easy—and I hated it. I hadn't gone off to war looking for easy. And even though Al Asad had an Echelon II medical facility, medically it wasn't very interesting, either.

The military command structure gets a little complicated, but basically there are three levels, or echelons, of medical facilities in a combat zone. Echelon I is a battalion aid station (BAS), a so-called "doc in a box," which takes care of routine medical problems for a battalion of about six hundred personnel. A BAS is staffed with a general medical officer (GMO) and corpsmen, but it has no surgical capability. The GMO is typically a very young doc who has just finished an internship and handles physicals and daily sick call. An Echelon II facility, meanwhile, has a surgical team with at least two surgeons, an anesthesiologist, nurses, and OR techs. Its job is to stabilize seriously wounded patients—stop the bleeding, get the blood pressure and breathing to survivable levels, perform basic surgery, sometimes called "meatball" surgery—and then get them ready for transport, usually by air, to an Echelon III facility for further treatment. An Echelon III facility is a field hospital like the kind portrayed in the TV series *M*A*S*H*, although they are now called a Combat Support Hospital, or CaSH. A CaSH has a full range of doctors—neurosurgeons, cardiothoracic surgeons, radiologists, everything—as well as sophisticated diagnostic equipment such as CT scanners. In 2005 there were only two CaSHs in Iraq, an Army CaSH in Baghdad and an Air Force CaSH in Balad.

Although Al Asad had an Echelon II facility, it wasn't catching many cases—and frankly, the people there weren't quite sure what to do with me. In more or less typical military fashion, no one had even known I was coming. The problem was compounded by the fact that even though I was supposed to be just another replacement surgeon, I was a Navy captain with far more trauma experience than anyone else on the surgical team. I guess the concern was that I would use my rank and experience to bigfoot them, to try to take over—although they needn't have worried. The commanding officer of the surgical facility in Al Asad was a general surgeon who had gone through my Navy trauma training program in Los Angeles, and although he hadn't done a trauma case since his residency, he had been a quick learner. He was also an excellent leader.

So after a couple of weeks at Al Asad, when I heard they were expecting heavy activity in the city of Fallujah, they let me fly down to Camp Fallujah, another sprawling Marine base outside the city of the same name, to see if I could help them out. It was much busier in Camp Fallujah than at Al Asad, but not nearly as busy as I was expecting. That was good news—but I still felt that my trauma skills and experience could be better used elsewhere.

Salvation came in the form of a Marine regimental surgeon, like me a Navy captain and another graduate of my NTTC course in Los Angeles. He flew into Camp Fallujah and told me that the battle with insurgents in the city of Ramadi was heating up and was about to get even more intense, which would mean more casualties. He desperately wanted to put together a Forward Resuscitative Surgical System (FRSS) team to be based there.

FRSS teams were the most forward-deployed surgical teams—that is, those most likely to get shot at—the Navy and Marines had. Small, with just two surgeons, two anesthesiologists, two OR corpsmen, and a critical-care nurse, they were designed to offer almost immediate surgical care to seriously wounded troops who, after being stabilized by the FRSS team, would then be medevac'ed to a higher-level facility in the rear. During the initial invasion of Iraq, the FRSS teams had been mobile, able to quickly pack up and advance with the front line, but as the war went static, with Marines and soldiers operating out of fixed bases in counterinsurgency warfare, the FRSS teams were more or less permanently planted in locations close to the fight.

I knew all about FRSS teams. Over the past eight years I had been deeply involved with other Navy medical personnel in their development, helping to determine their structure and equipment and personally testing their effectiveness during field exercises with the Marines. A lot of senior admirals and Navy medical officers thought we were nuts to take a surgical team so close to the fighting, but I couldn't think of anything I wanted to do more than put together an FRSS team and take it into combat.

It took me about a week to assemble the team. There was a Navy general surgeon who was two years out of his residency, and who for reasons I'll explain later we called J.C. There were two US Army "gas passers"—an anesthesiologist and a CRNA, or certified registered nurse anesthetist—one of whom we called Slipper Boy because he was always wearing slippers, and another we called Robusto for his love of cigars. There was a female critical-care nurse whose job was to accompany patients on the helicopters when they were medevac'ed out. She was a mature, good-looking, enthusiastic woman we called Blue Light Special because she carried a blue-lensed tactical Mini Mag flashlight, which some people say is better at illuminating blood in the dark than the red-lensed ones. Two Navy corpsmen served as OR techs. I was head surgeon and unit commander, and in rank, age, and experience was by far the most senior member of the team.

I also had to assemble our unit's AMAL—Authorized Medical Allowance List (everything has to have an acronym)—which was all the medical gear the team would need, or at least all that we were allowed: a portable oxygen generator, two three-kilowatt electrical generators, portable operating tables with lights, a portable anesthesia vaporizer and portable ventilators, monitors for blood pressure, temperature, electrocardiography, and on and on. It all got loaded onto a CH-46 helicopter and off we went to our new home—Camp Ramadi.

At the time, Ramadi was considered one of the most dangerous places in Iraq, with the entire city infested with insurgents. Heavily defended US outposts were placed in and around the city, and every patrol outside the wire stood a good chance of making contact with an ambush or IEDs (improvised explosive devices, so-called "roadside bombs"). Camp Ramadi was a collection of plywood huts, tents, and old Iraqi buildings situated on the outskirts of the city near the Euphrates River. There was a pretty good D-FAC (dining facility or chow hall) and there were shower trailers with toilets, but the Porta-Johns were much closer. From the air it looked like a shantytown—a shantytown equipped with hundreds of military vehicles, bristling with communications antennas, and covered with piles of sandbags and lines of Hesco boxes, which were wire-mesh-and-cardboard boxes that could be filled with dirt and stacked up to stop blast fragments.

An American artillery unit was based nearby, and I quickly learned the difference between the reassuring sound and concussive feel of outgoing artillery rounds, which I had felt before, and the distinctly unreassuring sound and feel of incoming enemy mortar rounds and rockets, which I hadn't felt before. A private who saw me looking around bewildered after a particularly loud boom explained it this way: "Sir, when you feel it in your feet, it's incoming artillery. If you feel it in your chest, it's outgoing." This was useful information.

Fortunately, the local bad guys were notoriously poor shots; they would point a mortar tube in the general direction of the camp, drop a few rounds, and then run away. Barring a direct hit, we were pretty safe behind our sandbags and Hesco boxes. If there was a direct hit—well, that's why they paid us the big bucks.

Although Ramadi was at the time generally a Marine show, there were a number of Army units operating there under command of Marine II MEF. Our Navy surgical unit was attached to the 228th Forward Support Battalion of the Pennsylvania Army National Guard, and more specifically to the 228th's "C" or "Charlie" Company, which was a medical company, and thus "Charlie Med." Charlie Med had about seventy personnel, including an emergency room doctor, two physician's assistants, and about fifty Army medics and ambulance drivers, along with administrative staff. Before we showed up, Charlie Med was an Echelon I facility; with the arrival of our surgical team, it was now effectively Echelon II.

(I also had a medical-support role to play for a US special operations team that was operating in Ramadi, targeting and capturing—or, more often, terminating—certain "high value" targets among the insurgents. As the old joke goes, I could tell you more about the special ops guys' missions, but then I'd have to kill you.)

The Army National Guard guys we were attached to were "citizen" soldiers, meaning that when they weren't on active military duty they had jobs in the civilian world—which means they were a pretty eclectic bunch. Of Charlie Med's administrative staff, Charlie's company commander, a huge, tall, thin, bald guy known affectionately as Bear, was a game warden by trade, while the executive officer, the XO, was a short guy who worked in a county coroner's office. The senior enlisted man, the first sergeant, known as Top, was a retired small-town police chief. On the medical side, the ER doctor was a thin, older family practitioner who had somehow managed to pass the Army physical. The ambulance platoon leader was a shy, quiet young woman who in civilian life was a kindergarten teacher. One of the physician's assistants was an instructor at Seton Hall.

Naturally, the first thing I wanted to see when we arrived was what was intended to be our operating room—a fifteen-by-thirty-foot unused plywood shack next to Charlie Med's battalion aid station. I was pleased to see that the floor had a smooth laminated surface, which was a step up from dirt or concrete, and meant that it could be mopped and kept reasonably clean. But the rest of it was a mess, every surface covered with an eighth-inch layer of dust.

A word here about dust in Iraq. Although Iraq was sometimes referred to as the Sandbox, sand really had nothing to do with it, at least not in the Euphrates and Tigris river valleys. The dirt there was alluvial silt that had been deposited over the aeons, and when it was dry it was like talcum powder; every footstep raised little puffs of dust, and vehicles would churn up clouds of the stuff. When the dust storms known as haboobs would kick up, the air would turn a weird orange color and visibility would be about ten feet. When it rained, the dust would turn into mud with the consistency of peanut butter.

As you can imagine, it's impossible to maintain a sterile OR in that kind of environment, although we tried as best we could. We washed and scrubbed the floors, walls, and ceiling of our plywood operating room repeatedly, sealed the cracks and joints in the plywood with rolls and rolls of duct tape, then put up two layers of blankets as curtains in the corridor between the makeshift ER and the prep room and the OR. After a week of constant scrubbing, the built-up dirt in the plywood came off and the OR started to stay clean, with only light dust getting on the equipment and supplies. It wasn't exactly sterile, but it was better than operating in a tent with dirt floors. Every day I would come in after my techs had cleaned everything and I would run my fingers over the surfaces, looking for areas that they missed. They hated that, but it had to be done.

But even before we had a chance to shape up the OR, while we were still unpacking our medical gear and setting up, we got our first casualty—brought to us in, of all things, a white BMW sedan.

It was a middle-aged Iraqi woman who had suffered multiple gunshot wounds from a .50-caliber machine gun—one of our machine guns. The story was that she had been charging at a TCP (traffic control point) in her car, and the Army sentries on duty had gone through the escalating levels of force required by the rules of engagement (ROEs): warning shot, then shoot the tires, then the engine block, then into the passenger compartment. That was the story, anyway. But in actual practice it may not have happened that way. Often there simply wasn't time to go through all those steps. Our troops had been getting hit with a lot of VBIEDs (vehicle-borne improvised explosive devices), cars or trucks packed with explosives, and it was a lot to ask young soldiers to strictly follow the ROEs and risk being blown to bits when a car was speeding toward them.

However it actually went down, they shot the woman and then rushed her over to us. The rule on treating Iraqis was that if we shot them, we treated them, even if they were EPWs (enemy prisoners of war). We also treated Iraqis who were working with us as Iraqi police or army soldiers, as well as any other Iraqi civilians who were brought to us. Basically our policy was, You bring 'em and we treat 'em.

As for the wounded EPWs, they got the same medical treatment that any of our wounded guys got—no more, no less. That was the rule, legally and morally, and I insisted on it being followed by everyone on the Charlie Med staff, no matter what emotions they might have had. Once, later in my deployment, we got three critical patients in—one a little girl hit in the head by an IED bomb fragment, another a Marine who was shot by a sniper when he was rescuing the little girl, and the other the insurgent sniper who had shot the Marine and was then shot by other Marines. And some of the young medics started muttering, "Hey, why are we even treating this son of a bitch? He shot our guy!" All three of the casualties made it, but later I gave the medics a little "motivational" talk—actually it was a pretty comprehensive ass-chewing—about how they were lucky to be serving a country that demanded humane treatment for everyone, and that everyone who came to us would be treated the same. I made it clear that those enemy combatants were first and foremost human beings, even though they'd had the misfortune to be born on the wrong side. I also made it clear that if I ever even suspected they weren't giving a 100 percent effort on everyone, I would personally make sure that they would be sorry they had ever been born—or words to that effect. They were good kids, but they just needed a little direction on our mission and where their duty lay. I never heard any muttering about treating EPWs after that.

Anyway, they brought the poor woman who'd been shot at the roadblock to us, and it was amazing that she was still alive. I'd seen thousands of bullet wounds before in civilian trauma centers, but not even the Crips and Bloods had .50-caliber weapons, which fire bullets that are a half inch in diameter at their widest point and can cause almost unbelievable damage to a human body. The weapon was designed to take out buildings and vehicles and aircraft, not necessarily people. It struck me at that moment that trauma surgery in the combat zone was going to be different from the usual day at a civilian trauma center.

One of the fifty-cals had pretty much blown the woman's left arm off above the elbow, leaving a gaping orange-sized hole where skin, muscle, and bone once had been. She had also been shot in the chest and abdomen several times and several times in her right leg. The leg was mush, the bones all broken. I had never seen a person so extensively damaged by gunfire, at least not one who was still alive. We took her directly from the vehicle to the OR.

We intubated her and put her out, then started working on her. As it turned out, we had four surgeons available that day. In addition to J.C. and me, there were an Air Force general surgeon and an Air Force orthopedic surgeon, both assigned to the aforementioned special ops team, although they would soon be shipping out to another assignment.

I told the Air Force surgeons to control the profuse bleeding from the arterial squirter in her arm, and J.C. and I started on her torso. We put two large tubes into her chest to drain blood and air and stop the bleeding from the lungs and chest. Then we dove into her belly, where it seemed like just about every organ was shot up. Her spleen was removed and went into a bucket in about one minute. Her liver was bleeding profusely, so we packed the area around it as tight as we could with sponges to stop the bleeding, then concentrated on controlling the bleeding from her intestines. We cut out sections of intestines and colon and then did damage-control surgery. It was pure meatball surgery, just trying to control the bleeding and contamination; the finesse work could be done later. Our job was to do the absolute bare minimum to keep her alive so that we could fly her to Baghdad or Balad, where there was a real field hospital. When we zipped her belly shut we only sutured the skin instead of closing the belly muscles, since the surgeons in Baghdad were going to have to open her up again anyway—assuming she survived the trip.

The Air Force guys were having trouble finding and controlling the bleeding from the big artery in her arm; there was a huge puddle of blood under their feet. I stepped in and cut the arm off high up near the shoulder with a scalpel and a pair of surgical scissors. This was wartime surgery; there wasn't time to try to save the arm. We could save her right leg, though, which was broken and badly mangled but with the blood flow still intact. Normally we would open up the leg and screw metal plates into the bone to hold it together, but again, this was combat surgery, so there wasn't time. We had brought an external fixator—an "ex-fix"—with us, which allowed us to quickly put screws into the bone and put on the bone-supporting metal brace externally to temporarily keep the bone in place until it could be permanently repaired. Then we packed her up and put her on a medevac flight to Baghdad.

I had been pleased with the results of our first casualty. Our forward surgical unit had worked exactly as it was designed to do: nothing fancy, just get the patient stabilized and passed along—true meatball surgery. Since we didn't have an ICU, or the staff and gear for one, it wasn't our job to provide long-term critical care. That was for the guys in Baghdad and Balad.

As it turned out, the Iraqi woman survived the medevac flight and was successfully treated at the Baghdad CaSH. A week later she was flown back to Ramadi and released to Iraqi medical authorities for treatment—or was supposed to be. Two months later we got an Iraqi civilian request for medical assistance for an unidentified injured woman, so we sent a medic out with a patrol to see her in her home. When the medic got back he told me, "Doc, you aren't going to believe this," and showed me a picture he'd taken of the patient. It was her, the lady from the white BMW, still wearing bandages from where we had taken off her arm. But what really hit me was the picture he had taken of her injured leg. She still had the ex-fix device screwed into her leg! The Iraqi doctors should have taken that out weeks earlier, but apparently they didn't realize that it was a temporary fix, not a permanent solution. I sent the medic back out to tell the woman's family to make sure an Iraqi doctor unscrewed the thing from her leg. I hope they did.

While we were getting settled in on the medical side, we also started improving our living conditions a little bit. There was an old shack on a concrete pad about the size of a tractor trailer near the surgical hut, so we tore it down and started building a sleeping "hooch." Top, the first sergeant, scrounged up some two-by-fours and some pallets of plywood, along with some hammers and saws and nail guns. A couple of the sergeants in the ambulance squad had been contractors back home, and it turned out that in addition to being a fine surgeon, J.C. was a pretty good carpenter—so good that we started calling him "J.C.," after another carpenter who lived a couple of millennia ago. We all set to work on it, and after about a week we had it done, managing not to saw off any of our extremities in the process. We divided the structure into three rooms, one for the female flight nurse, one for the chaplain, and one for me. We wired it for electricity, and I found an old door to use as a desk. I even managed to wire the hooch with Internet access. The military had its own secure and nonclassified Internet systems—known as SIPRNet and the NIPRNet—but the bandwidth was limited. But of course, being a National Guard company, Charlie Med had a medic who was a cable TV guy back home, and with a few hundred yards of "borrowed" wire he tapped into a civilian Internet system for me. The engineers also bulldozed a softball field in an open space behind Charlie Med, which was great except that the 'dozers left a lot of rocks and ridges that made for some dramatic bad hops on grounders. I played second base.

Not that we had a whole lot of downtime. When we weren't treating casualties, I insisted on putting the surgical team and the medics assigned to us through mass-casualty drills, over and over, learning how to manage a sudden influx of wounded, how to work together efficiently as a team. It didn't necessarily endear me to the troops, but it was necessary. Particularly important in mass-casualty situations is the triage stage—*triage* being French for "sorting out." Triaging was one of my jobs. During triage you assign the wounded to three basic categories: those who need surgery right now, those who can wait a little while, and those for whom no amount of surgery or care is going to do any good. These last are called "expectant." They are going to die.

It sounds simple enough, but it's not. How you perform triage depends on a host of factors. How many OR tables do you have? How many surgeons? How many OR packs are on hand? How many units of blood are available? Most significantly, how many wounded are coming in? If you've got only one casualty, it doesn't matter if you doubt he's going to survive; you get him into the OR and see what you can do. But if there are twenty serious casualties, you can't waste time and resources trying to save the doomed while letting others who stand a chance wait and die. At civilian trauma centers in the States, you always tried to do everything you could for everyone, but in Iraq, in the dirt, there was no way we had the gear and the people to do that. It makes for hard choices, but it's what you have to do. In the old days the military usually assigned the staff dental officer or a senior nurse or medic to conduct triage, but I always insisted that a surgeon make the calls on serious cases.

Fortunately, for the first month our casualties came in ones and twos—an Iraqi soldier shot in the left foot, a Marine shot in the side in the gap between his body armor who needed a resection of most of his bowels and stomach. (He survived, and three days later was at Bethesda Naval Hospital.)

One interesting thing was that the bullet wounds we were getting were far different from the bullet wounds we saw in the civilian world. Almost all of the gunshot wounds stateside were from handguns; very few were high-velocity rifle rounds. In Iraq it was the opposite, and the damaging effects on the human body were greatly increased. I'd had some experience with rifle bullet wounds; in fact, when I was in medical school they used to shoot anesthetized goats with rifle rounds to teach us on to deal with them, although when that got out the animal-rights people managed to get that practice stopped. But in Iraq I got a lot of experience in high-velocity bullet wounds.

Anyway, the first few weeks at Camp Ramadi were relatively easy. But then came Pearl Harbor Day.

As I said, it had started off pretty good, with those freshly cleaned and sanitized Porta-Johns. There'd been a Pearl Harbor memorial service at the camp—it seems like only World War II vets and the military remember the day anymore—and had remained pretty much routine until well after evening chow. Then someone knocked on my hooch door and called out, "Captain Rhee, urgent surgical Marines incoming!"

Marines. Plural. Not good—but not necessarily accurate, either. Sometimes we'd get alerted to stand by for multiple casualties and only one or even none would come in—which was never a disappointment. I ran out to the casualty drop-off area just outside the OR hut.

I started to get the story—a typical story in Ramadi and throughout Iraq. Marines in Humvees were on patrol when an IED went off, damaging one vehicle. The Marines dismounted to help their buddies and another IED went off, and then another. Eleven Marines were wounded, at least six critically; they were on the way to Charlie Med.

The first Humvee bearing casualties came screaming around the corner, horn blaring, and skidded to a panic stop. The medics pulled out a wounded Marine and put him on a stretcher, his mangled legs dangling off the side, and started running toward the OR. It was a natural reaction—a badly wounded man comes in, you rush him to the OR—but not the right one. I yelled for them to stop and put the stretcher on the deck until I could assess his condition. (I made a mental note to myself: more drills on this required.) Already I could hear more vehicles coming, bringing in more wounded. We couldn't tie up the OR with this Marine until we knew if he urgently needed it.

He did. He was bleeding badly from what was left of his legs, he was gasping for breath, like a fish dying on a riverbank, but there was no air exchange. Yep, he was urgent. I told the medics to take him to the OR and told the OR techs to have a retractor ready in case I had to open his chest. I asked Bear, the Charlie Med CO, to get a walking blood bank going—that is, start collecting blood from Charlie Med support troops and anyone else they could find. We were going to need blood and a lot of it. I headed into the OR.

The first wounded Marine, still on a stretcher, was on one of the two operating tables we had in the operating room, the stretcher resting on table brackets. We operated right on the stretchers, but a stretcher is like a hammock; it sags in the middle and causes your arms and shoulders to fold in. To prevent this, J.C. had built wooden contraptions that I designed that sat on the operating tables and raised the center of the body three inches as the stretcher was laid down, giving us better access to the chest. J.C.'s homemade devices were covered in duct tape and spray-painted red so the blood wouldn't show as much.

We started cutting off the Marine's body armor so we could check him for other wounds, but it wasn't easy. In a civilian trauma center the ER team will have a patient naked in less than fifteen seconds, but the armor vest and the ceramic SAPI (small arms protective inserts) inside it are heavy, about twenty-six pounds, and cutting through Kevlar fabric, even with surgical shears, takes effort. We finally got it off him. There were no wounds to his back or chest, which were fish-belly white (no sunbathing allowed for Marine grunts in Iraq). His face was black with soot, and he reeked with the kerosene smell of JP-8 fuel from the damaged Humvee.

The Marine had tourniquets high up on both legs, which were put on by the field corpsman who first got to him. Good. That action probably had saved his life for now. For years I and others had been battling the widely held notion among civilian surgeons that tourniquets did more harm than good, and we had finally succeeded in making tourniquets standard-issue for soldiers and Marines. True, a tourniquet that was improperly placed or left on for too long could cause complications, ranging from amputation to actual increased blood loss, but those problems were the result of lack of training, not the tourniquets themselves. The tourniquets on this Marine were a bit too loose, so I tightened them. I put a huge tube directly into his major vein in the groin and an A-line into the artery so that we could attach it to an arterial blood monitoring system that allowed us to continuously see what his blood pressure was. I told the OR tech to sew them into the groin so they wouldn't fall out. We started infusing one of ten units of red blood cells that we had in the refrigerator until the walking blood bank could start bringing in fresh whole blood. The anesthesiologist, Slipper Boy, told me he could feel a pulse.

J.C. ran into the OR and said he was bringing in another urgent casualty and there were five more urgents outside, two with double above-the-knee amputations, meaning that both legs were already blown completely off. I quickly amputated what was left of the first Marine's left leg, snipping through the scraps of flesh and tendons and clamping off arteries, and then I ran out to attend to the other casualties.

It was a surreal scene outside—pitch-dark, litters everywhere, wool Army blankets covering the wounded, the medics' and nurses' headband flashlights casting weird shadows everywhere. The Navy GMO assigned to the wounded Marines' unit was there, doing what he could, pushing blood through an IV into a Marine with a mangled left leg. Another casualty, one torn-up leg barely hanging from his hip, was conscious and talking to a PA. Two other casualties were double amputees, with only stumps at midthigh—amputations by IED. Tourniquets had stopped the bleeding—more lives saved by tourniquets—and their blood pressure was holding steady.

"How ya doin', Marine?" I asked one of them as I looked him over. He was conscious, the morphine injection the field corpsman gave him reducing some of the pain but still leaving him lucid; he knew he didn't have legs anymore.

"Fine, sir," he said in a whisper. "Go ahead and take care of someone else."

I would hear it a hundred times during my tour in Iraq from battle-mangled Marines and soldiers. "I'm fine, doc. Take care of my buddy. He's worse off than I am. Save him, save him."

Those kids. Those poor, brave, selfless, magnificent kids. They were always looking out for each other, always more worried about their buddies than they were about themselves. It wasn't something you often saw in the civilian world. I couldn't get emotional then, though. There was too much work to do.

I ran back into the OR, where J.C. was taking off one of the second casualty's legs at the thigh. One quick glance and I saw that his other leg looked bad as well, and probably should also have come off. But J.C. thought he could save it, so I didn't say anything. I had to give him room to work and let him make the call on what he needed to do. I went back to the first casualty, who was still on the OR table. He was stable, so we packed him for helicopter medevac to the Echelon III CaSH in Baghdad.

Packing patients for air medevac was different than in the civilian world. The Army used dedicated medical helicopters, Black Hawks that were specifically configured to transport patients, while the Marines provided air-evac helicopters on an as-available basis, usually CH-46s. In either case the winter air blowing through the cargo/passenger compartment could be bitterly cold—and cold was our badly wounded patients' mortal enemy. So to keep them warm during the flight we would wrap them first in a wool blanket, then in a space-age reflective thermal blanket, and then in a zipped-up body bag—yes, the same kind of body bag we used for the dead, except with a hole cut out for the face. The lifesaving IV lines and chest tube lines and breathing tubes and the wires for the monitors all came out the same hole, with the monitoring equipment resting on top of the patient on the stretcher.

I decided to send the double amputees out on the same chopper, without operating on them. It wouldn't have done any good to operate on them at our level; their bleeding was controlled with the tourniquets and we didn't have the time. If we did operate we would have had to intubate them, which could complicate things on the flight to Baghdad. The chopper came into the LZ (landing zone) nearby, the patients were loaded aboard with medics and a flight nurse to monitor them en route, and off they went.

The Navy GMO called out to me, saying his patient was crashing. He was conscious and the GMO was giving him blood, but he couldn't keep up. He was losing him. I knew he must still be bleeding. We got him on the newly vacated OR table and I saw that he was unresponsive and going down fast. The surgical symphony we had practiced and performed so many times began: tube in the trachea, lines go in, left leg comes off, fresh blood that was now available from the walking blood bank goes in. The battalion chaplain and the motor pool first sergeant were helping Robusto, the CRNA, squeeze donated blood into the patient. The fresh whole blood had come directly from the arm of a soldier a hundred feet away, and after being checked for compatibility it was pushed, still warm, into the patient. It was lifesaving, far better than the refrigerated stuff we used at home.

I took the tourniquet off the Marine's right leg and used the Doppler stethoscope to check for pulses in the right foot. The

Doppler was finicky—sometimes it seemed like you had to stand on one leg and hold the earphone jack upside down to make the damn thing work—but finally I heard the whish-whish-whish sounds that spelled good news. Blood was flowing. The Marine had lost one leg, but the other leg had a chance. We wrapped him up, bound for Baghdad.

Outside the OR it was still a scene of controlled chaos. Officers and NCOs from the wounded Marines' unit had shown up to check on their men; they were standing around looking like worried parents. The line of soldiers waiting to give blood snaked around the building, probably a hundred of them. By that time we had told them that we had run out of blood bags to collect their blood, but they wouldn't leave, just in case.

I had called in another medevac helicopter to pick up our second batch of casualties; it was due in about ten minutes. All of the wounded were stabilized. But suddenly there was a flurry of activity around J.C.'s first patient, who was now wrapped and waiting for medevac. His oxygen saturation level was dropping; J.C. wasn't getting a reading on the pulse oximeter. The saturation drop told me he was losing blood and his blood pressure was plummeting. We peeled away the packing layers—body bag, thermal blanket, Army blanket—and, yep, there it was, a pool of blood collecting in the bottom of the bag, coming from the Marine's remaining mangled leg. At the bottom of the leg there was half a foot, in half a boot.

J.C. knew he had made a mistake. When he was helping to pull the wounded Marine out of the Humvee, the Marine, a young, muscular, athletic type, had wrapped his arms around J.C.'s neck and pleaded with him to save his legs. In those few seconds J.C. had formed an emotional connection to the man— the kind of connection that a surgeon can't afford to have in a mass trauma situation. He hadn't been able to bring himself to take off that second leg, hoping that the orthopedic docs in Baghdad could save it. It was the wrong call and could have cost this young Marine his life.

"We gotta take the leg, J.C.," I told him—and we had to do it fast. The chopper had arrived, and if the Marine didn't get on it he would die here. We didn't have the ICU capability to keep him alive for long. J.C. knew I was right, and we proceeded to take off the leg at the thigh, definitively controlling his bleeding while our anesthesia guys continued to pump precious fresh blood into him. In ten minutes we were done. We gave him the seventh unit of blood, repacked him, and got him to the bird just in time.

And then, suddenly, it was eerily quiet at Charlie Med. All of the casualties had been evacuated. Two hours had gone by since the first casualty had come in. It felt like it had been only minutes, and at the same time it felt like it had been days. It was late, everybody was exhausted, and most had gone to bed. I called a debrief for the medical staff, but it was about two in the morning so I heard the groans. They were thinking I was going to chew them out for whatever had gone wrong tonight. But that wasn't what I had in mind.

"In military medicine there is no greater honor or privilege than the opportunity to serve the men and women of the armed forces in wartime," I told them when they had assembled. "To make a difference in the field is the ultimate reward. What happened tonight is something you will always remember. If you are not affected by it, then you don't understand what just happened, and you don't have a heart. What Charlie Med did tonight was save lives and limbs. You did a great job. Hooah for Charlie Med! Dismissed!"

I meant every word of it. I was proud of those young men and women.

The day had gone about as well as could reasonably have been expected. The mass-casualty drills had paid off; we had worked well together as a team. Back in my hooch I started writing up the paperwork—actually, the computer work—on our casualties. Every US casualty in Iraq and Afghanistan was documented and tracked so that we could statistically assess what worked and what hadn't and how we could improve things. On this day, Pearl Harbor Day, we had treated eleven Marines, six of whom had serious leg injuries. Of the twelve legs on those six Marines, four had been missing when they arrived at Charlie Med, we took off three in the OR, and four more were taken off in Baghdad. We saved only one out of the twelve legs.

There was a knock on the door, and J.C. came in and sat on a folding chair with his head in his hands. He was still bothered by the Marine he'd almost lost, the one we found bleeding out while he was packed and waiting for the chopper. J.C. had done civilian trauma work during his residency, had seen some gangbanger-style shooting cases, but he'd never seen anything like this, never seen so many young men broken and torn while fighting for their country. He knew he should have taken the other leg off, but he had desperately wanted to help that young Marine keep at least one of his legs. His emotions had outweighed his medical judgment, and he knew it.

I let him talk. It was good for him to get it out. If he hadn't had a heart he would have had no business being in this business, but he had learned a hard lesson that night. I had learned some things, too. I'd had a lot of trauma experience, but this was my first combat mass casualty in a war zone. I knew I would never forget this day—and I never have.

After J.C. left I waited up for Blue Light Special, the flight nurse who had accompanied the first chopper to Baghdad, to get back. She finally got back at 0400, and I asked how the medevac flight went.

She waved me off and said, "Captain, let me go brush my teeth first."

When she got back she explained that during the flight a medic had discovered that one of the double amputees wasn't breathing, even though he'd been stable when they'd put him on the bird. So Blue Light, weighed down with about fifty pounds of body armor and other gear, had started doing chest compressions and giving him epinephrine injections and giving him mouth-to-mouth resuscitation in the freezing cold until they got to Baghdad. His lips and face were still covered in battle grime, and while she was giving the dying Marine CPR he had vomited into her mouth. That was why she had wanted to brush her teeth.

We later found out that when the medics were loading the legless Marine onto the Army Blackhawk in the dark, with the rotor blades kicking up dust and everyone trying desperately to hurry, his IV line had gotten snagged and broken off. Once the bird was airborne, still in the dark, with the wind whipping through the open door windows at a hundred miles per hour, no one noticed that he was bleeding out backward from the cut IV line until he stopped breathing.

Blue Light was heartsick about it; her hands were trembling as she talked to me. But she was hopeful.

"I got him back," she told me. "I think he had a pulse when I handed him off at the CaSH."

But it wasn't enough. I soon found out that that young Marine died of blood loss shortly after arriving in Baghdad.

The Marine's death would be officially listed by me as "preventable"—the only such death I would have in Iraq. It would mean more training, more drills, more work to guard against the unexpected and the unforeseen. We would do everything humanly possible to prevent more "preventable" deaths.

And yet in a war zone that term somehow seems out of place,

almost meaningless. In war, young men and women live or die by the smallest of margins—a step to the left instead of the right, an IED detonated a tenth of a second sooner or later, an IV line caught in a rotor wash and snagged on a chopper door. You could argue that every death in war is preventable. We could prevent them all if somehow we could just not have any wars.

After Blue Light left I stayed up for a while longer, until I knew I could fall into a dead sleep without thinking too much. I slept for a few hours and then went outside—and this time it wasn't so early in the morning, and there were no "fresh" Porta-Johns.

A few hours later I was in my office hooch and there was a knock on the door.

"Captain Rhee? We've got four more coming in . . ."

It went on like that in the following weeks. Marines and soldiers and Iraqis coming in, mostly by ones and two and threes, with bullet wounds from firefights, fragmentation wounds from IEDs, backs broken from flipped-over Humvees, fingers and hands amputated by getting caught in the tracks of tanks or armored personnel carriers—every kind of terrible wound that war can produce. We were doing chest surgery, belly surgery, vascular surgery, and a lot of urologic surgery, as the area around the groin was unprotected by body armor except for a light Kevlar flap. A lot of young Marines and soldiers were getting shot down there, or blown up with injuries to the groin. Not a pretty picture.

Sometimes Marines or soldiers would come in who should have been dead but weren't. I remember one night we had two guys come in, one Marine and one Army soldier, both shot in the head by a sniper, the AK-47 high-velocity bullets hitting them squarely in the front of their Kevlar helmets. Kevlar will not stop an AK-47 round. Almost miraculously, in both cases the rounds had carved huge gashes in their scalps but hadn't penetrated their skulls. Those were the two luckiest guys in Iraq that day.

We had been lucky, too. When they came in by ones or twos or threes J.C. and I could easily handle them; even the eleven Marines brought in on Pearl Harbor Day, six of them critical, hadn't overwhelmed us.

But that changed on another day—January 5, 2006, what we would always remember as Rose Bowl Day.

We had just finished watching Texas beat USC over our jury-rigged TV when the word came in: incoming mass casualties, maybe a dozen. That proved to be a massive underestimate.

It turned out that a suicide bomber wearing an explosive vest had walked into an Iraqi police recruiting center that had been set up in a glass factory not far beyond the Camp Ramadi perimeter; about five hundred Iraqis had shown up to try to get police jobs. Some Marine K-9 dog handlers were helping to provide security for the event, and when one of them approached the suicide bomber, he detonated the device packed with ball bearings and forty pounds of explosives. When the smoke and dust cleared, the suicide bomber's guts were splattered against a wall and his torso—just his torso—was lying in the dirt. Around him dozens of people were dead and hundreds were wounded by blast and shrapnel, almost all of them Iraqis. It was the bloodiest suicide attack since the war had started.

At Charlie Med we had drilled over and over for mass casualties—which to me at the time meant ten, twenty, even thirty. But this was something new.

I called in everybody—on-duty, off-duty, everybody—and ordered another walking blood bank to get started. I ran out to the receiving area just as the first casualty came in the back of a white Mercedes sedan that had been commandeered as an ambulance. It was a young Marine sergeant. As I examined him

I couldn't find any obvious wounds, but he wasn't breathing and had no palpable pulse. He was dead.

Now I had a hard choice to make.

If the dead Marine had been the only casualty, I would have sent him to the OR and opened him up and tried to bring him back. It probably wouldn't have worked, but I would have tried anyway.

But as I was bent over the dead Marine I could see and hear the other casualties coming in, in Humvees and ambulances and private Iraqi vehicles and even in a dump truck. I knew there would be dozens of critically injured people in them, people who were still alive and could be saved. Could I tie up one of our two OR tables and use up precious blood and surgical supplies on this deceased Marine when there were others who could be saved?

I said before it was a hard choice, and, yes, for me as a human being it was hard emotionally. But medically, as a trauma surgeon doing mass-casualty triage, it wasn't a difficult choice. In fact, it was no choice at all. Again, it's what mass-casualty triage is all about. You save the ones who can be saved and have to leave the certain-to-die to their fate.

Quietly, so the other Marines standing nearby couldn't hear, I told a medic to take the young Marine to the expectant area, the place where we kept the dead and the soon to be dead. I told him to make doubly certain that the Marine was dead there because I didn't have the time to wait and confirm it. The medic got into the vehicle and told the driver to start moving. As they took the young Marine away I couldn't help wondering if I'd done the right thing. My head told me I had, but my heart wasn't sure. What if in the heat of the moment I had simply missed the pulse? What if that young Marine actually was still alive? But I didn't have time to dwell on it.

Later I learned that the Marine sergeant was the dog handler who had first approached the suicide bomber. Apparently the suicide bomber's body had shielded him from shrapnel, but the concussion of the blast had caused massive internal injuries that had killed him almost instantly without leaving any external wounds. His K-9 dog was hit by shrapnel but survived.

I had made the right call, but that didn't make it any easier. And it wasn't the last time that day that I had to make a decision like that.

As I ran from vehicle to vehicle, some of them packed with a half dozen or a dozen wounded, I would loudly call out, "How are you?" I knew that the wounded who responded could wait; the others needed immediate attention. Some of the wounds were ghastly; several of the wounded had pieces of human bone lodged in them—not their own bone, but bone shards from other victims who had been blown apart in the blast.

And many of the wounds were hopeless—brain matter hanging out, multiple limbs sheared off, bellies eviscerated. Or at least they were hopeless in Camp Ramadi. If it had been LA instead of Iraq, if we had had eight surgeons and a dozen ORs and all the supplies in the world, we might have been able to save some of them. But it wasn't. It was the combat zone, and we were being overwhelmed. There were so many wounded that as we lifted them out of the vehicles we had to lay them down in the dirt road because we had run out of stretchers.

So eleven more times that day I had to look into the faces of wounded men, all of them Iraqis, and decide that there was no hope, that other savable patients would have to come first, and that the wounded man would have to be taken to the expectant area to die so that others could live.

I remember one of them distinctly still. He was a thin Iraqi man, probably in his early twenties, with a heavy dark beard and dried, cracked lips, dressed in a ragged shirt with worn sandals on his feet. His face was covered with dirt. Unusually for an Iraqi, his eyes were sky blue, and the clarity in them was profound. He was lying there in the dirt, propped up on his left elbow, and he was reaching up for me with his right arm, his eyes begging me for help. As I knelt down to see what his injuries were he grabbed at my sleeve, pulling me closer, still looking at me with those clear blue eyes. As I tore my eyes away from his I saw a huge, gaping, bleeding hole in the left side of his head that had left brain matter exposed—a hopeless, mortal wound. When I looked back at his eyes I could see that he understood. I pulled his right hand from my sleeve and stood up. I looked around the massive number of bodies on the ground and spotted a medic a few feet away. I pointed to the man on the ground and yelled to the medic one word—"Expectant!" Then I had to move on to the next patient.

I've never forgotten that man's face, and the way his eyes locked on mine. I probably never will.

All told we handled more than seventy wounded that day, with dozens of others wounded in the suicide bombing being flown to Fallujah or Al Asad for treatment. The total death count from the bombing was fifty-eight people, including the Marine dog handler, an Army National Guard lieutenant colonel who died at the bombing scene, and the eleven Iraqis I had to declare expectant. All of the other wounded we treated survived.

It was the worst mass-casualty situation I had ever experienced, before or since. I had never had to declare a dozen people expectant, and I hope I never have to again. And it changed the way I look at mass-casualty medicine. I realized that in the civilian world as well as the military world, you can't train and prepare for what you think is going to happen—that is, ten or twenty or even thirty casualties coming in at the same time. To be ready, you have to train and be prepared for what you think is *never* going to happen—a hundred or two hundred or three hundred casualties at the same time. If you do that, you'll be ready for whatever comes up—including, for example, nineteen innocent people shot down by a madman in Tucson.

I finally finished my Iraq tour in March 2006. I left Charlie Med and came home with a feeling of satisfaction. I felt that I had at least partly paid back the Navy and my country for the time and money they had spent on my medical training. I had seen a lot and learned a lot that would help me in the world of civilian trauma and mass casualties. I believe we saved a lot of lives—and to the families of the ones we couldn't save, I can only say I'm truly sorry. I wish we had done better.

Some days at Charlie Med had been worse than others— Pearl Harbor Day, Rose Bowl Day. But every day that some broken and bloody American Marine or soldier or Iraqi civilian came in to Charlie Med was a bad day. And yet the fact that we were able to help so many injured people also made them good days.

So I guess the best way to sum it up is this:

Every day was a good bad day at Charlie Med.

CHAPTER 8

LAB WARS

I always felt bad for the pigs.

Pigs are supposedly one of the top ten smartest creatures in the animal world, on average much smarter than dogs, and their internal anatomy and physiology is very close to humans'. Which is why, when I was conducting medical research experiments on them, I always tried to keep two things in mind:

One was that we humans kill roughly three billion pigs a year to make bacon, ham, and pork chops.

And the other was that by sacrificing the lives of a few hundred pigs in medical research experiments, I was potentially helping to save the lives of thousands of human beings.

Medical research is an important part of being an academic surgeon. I mentioned earlier that when I was interviewing with the chairman of surgery at UC Irvine, he told me that he didn't want to produce merely competent clinical surgeons in his residency program—that his residency spots were for surgeons who wanted to be academicians, that he wanted to develop surgeons who would expand the profession, develop new and better ways of doing things.

At the time I didn't really understand what he meant, but after getting some experience in trauma surgery I did. I realized that there were basically two ways of working as a trauma surgeon, or as any kind of doctor. You could stay on the safe, paved roads of established medical knowledge, doing things a certain way because that's the way everybody did them. The other way was to get off the paved roads and blaze a new trail for others.

I decided I wanted to look for new trails. And to do that, to find new and better ways of doing things—and even more important, to convince other surgeons that the new ways were better—I had to spend time in the lab.

I was particularly interested in the field of trauma immunology, how traumatic injuries affect the human immune system, and as a resident at UCI, I had helped with a number of research projects on the subject using rats as test animals. But it wasn't until I was in the Washington, DC, area in the mid-1990s that I finally got a chance to strike out on my own.

Although I was working full-time as an attending trauma surgeon at Washington Hospital Center, and was also an assistant professor of surgery at my alma mater, the Uniformed Services University of the Health Sciences in Bethesda, I was young and ambitious enough to think that my plate still wasn't quite full. So I applied for and received a five-year grant from the Office of Naval Research to set up my own laboratory and conduct research into various aspects of trauma immunology.

Now, when people think of a research lab they usually envision a large, brightly lit, white-walled room with dozens of highly trained doctors and scientists in lab coats peering into microscopes and hovering over tubes and beakers, surrounded by gleaming state-of-the-art equipment. Maybe labs funded by giant pharmaceutical companies or that are receiving hundred-million-dollar grants are like that.

But I was working with limited funds, so my lab was a little different. After a lot of wrangling, I finally got the university to give me a small room deep in the basement of the main building that had once been used as a mock operating room to train medical students about OR procedures. My equipment was all stuff that I borrowed or bought secondhand or jury-rigged like something out of a *MacGyver* episode. And my research budget didn't quite cover hiring dozens of doctors and scientists. Instead, initially I could just barely afford to hire three lab techs, none of whom was a trained researcher or medical person. Solin was a college marine biology major, Brenda was planning to go to veterinary school, and Sylvester was a government employee who handled the animals and generally took care of the lab. They were all good people, but they didn't have medical experience—which meant that until I could teach them how to do things, I had to do almost all of the medical work myself, from administering anesthesia to operating the cardio-bypass pump.

Later I was lucky to hire Dr. Leon Sun, who had been a heart transplant surgeon in his native China, but who after immigrating to the US had to content himself with working as a research scientist. Dr. Sun had a heavy accent, but his written English was very good, and he was a top-notch editor of my research manuscripts. Although he wasn't licensed as a surgeon in the US, he was a thoroughly competent surgeon and a great help to me. Later still I was fortunate to find Dr. Hasan Alam, a young, Pakistan-born surgery resident at Washington Hospital Center who had gone through his trauma rotation at the hospital and was an excellent surgeon. Hasan was supposed to return to Pakistan after he finished his surgical training because his visa was expiring, but instead I persuaded him to come work for me in my lab while I got his visa issue straightened out. Hasan turned out to be a key player in my life, as I think I was in his. Later, at age forty-two, Hasan became one of the youngest full professors of surgery at Harvard Medical School.

So anyway, given the funding limitations, and the fact that I was already working two other jobs, my early days in the research lab were tough going. And yet I loved it. I think I learned more about medicine and surgery in those first five years of lab work than I ever did in medical school or even during residency.

Partly through hard work and partly through luck, my research made some contributions to medical knowledge and treatment.

One of those involved a condition known as Da Nang lung.

For decades the prevailing notion in medicine was that if a patient had extreme low blood pressure as a result of blood loss, you would pump him full of fluids to get the blood pressure back up, a process known as "fluid resuscitation"; the usual fluid was something called lactated Ringer's solution, which had been around since the nineteenth century. Sometimes the amount of fluid infusions was massive, as much as seventy liters a day. The medical community was convinced that the fluid infusions were saving lives, that without them the patient would surely die.

But there was one problem. After surviving the traumatic blood loss, patients who had received massive fluid infusions were later dying from inflammation and swelling of the organs—particularly the lungs. The patient's lungs would stiffen and fill up with water, and eventually the patient would die of respiratory failure. (Renal or kidney failure was another frequent post-traumatic cause of death.)

This lung condition was first noticed in the Vietnam War, when a lot of wounded soldiers were being treated with fluid resuscitations, only to develop lung problems and die. Doctors who worked at the Navy Field Hospital in Da Nang started calling it Da Nang lung because it affected so many patients there, but it was also called shock lung, stiff lung, and a host of other names. Later it was named Acute Respiratory Distress Syndrome, or ARDS. And for a long time ARDS was a major cause of postoperative death in trauma patients, both military and civilian.

I had seen it often. A patient with severe bleeding injuries would come into the trauma center and we'd get the blood pressure back up with fluid resuscitation and repair the damage and send him to the ICU. But even though we had fixed his injuries, he would start to die from all the internal inflammation. It was incredibly frustrating for us—and for the patient, it was all too often fatal.

The medical establishment came up with all sorts of explanations for what was causing ARDS and other post-traumatic internal swelling and inflammation—that it was the natural reaction of blood-deprived tissues being reoxygenated, that it was the inevitable result of medical advances that were allowing trauma patients to survive for longer periods and thus giving them time to develop the condition. Millions of research dollars and thousands of man-hours were being spent trying to figure out how to treat ARDS after patients developed it.

Early on in my career I too had been involved in related research, serving as the principal investigator in a multicenter study that was attempting to determine if a man-made monoclonal antibody could prevent this destructive inflammatory process in trauma patients. It was an extremely difficult study to conduct, not least because the patients we were testing it on were too injured to give their consent to be part of the research study, which meant we had to obtain consent from their family members. As you can imagine, the last thing someone whose loved one has been seriously injured wants to think about is signing a consent form for a medical research study. That's a persistent problem in any kind of trauma research on human subjects. And even when I could get the consent, I had to get the patient's blood sample on a private jet and fly it to a laboratory within four hours of obtaining it. It was pretty hectic.

In any event, after participating in that research, and after reading and listening to dozens and dozens of studies and presentations on the subject, I started thinking that maybe the medical establishment was going at it the wrong way. Instead of figuring out how to treat ARDS, I wanted to figure out what was causing ARDS in the first place. It occurred to me that maybe the resuscitative fluids we were pumping into hemorrhaging patients could be the problem. So in my little underfunded lab in the basement of the university building I started doing some experiments.

Which brings us back to the pigs.

Medical experiments on animals are a touchy subject. Primates such as monkeys are the closest creatures to humans, and thus would be the best research subjects. But that's the problem, they're too close to humans, and so for social and political reasons they are not readily accessible for scientific experiments. For approximating the internal anatomy and physiology of humans, pigs are the next best thing.

Of course, there are many regulatory checks and balances on large-animal medical research. Despite what some animal-rights activists may think, medical researchers want to make absolutely certain they are not inadvertently harming or hurting animals during their research. Which is why every research facility has a lab-animal review board that goes over every aspect of every proposed research project, down to making sure that the needles used to sedate the animals are the smallest size possible. Still, sometimes it weighs on my conscience.

For my major fluid-resuscitation experiments I used man-sized—about 150 pounds—Yorkshire pigs raised in a special lab-animal farm in Maryland. After getting preapproval from the university lab-animal review board, I anesthetized the pigs and drained 40 percent of their blood, putting them into hemorrhagic shock. I also had a control group in which I did not bleed the animals. Then I gave them infusions of various kinds of resuscitative fluids: lactated Ringer's solution, which was the accepted method; hypertonic saline solution; and the whole blood that I had removed from the pigs. What I found was that fresh blood was the best resuscitative fluid, hypertonic saline was the next best, and lactated Ringer's solution was the worst. In fact, when given in massive quantities, lactated Ringer's solution was actually causing conditions like ARDS.

To put it another way, while trying to save people's lives by giving them large infusions of those fluids, we were actually poisoning them.

Obviously, I'm greatly simplifying this process here. It's not like you do one set of experiments on a few pigs and suddenly throw up your arms and shout "Eureka!" It takes years, and dozens or even hundreds of experiments, before you can start drawing sound conclusions. You do one experiment for this, another for that, building up your evidence incrementally. And along the way you publish peer-reviewed papers to support your findings. I authored or coauthored some forty papers on the effects of resuscitative fluids, papers with titles that only a scientist would find exciting, such as "Lactated Ringer's Solution Resuscitation Causes Neutrophil Activation After Hemorrhagic Shock" and "Resuscitation-Induced Pulmonary Apoptosis and Intracellular Adhesion Molecule-1 Expression Are Attenuated by the Use of Ketone Ringer's Solution." It was all incredibly complicated. There was also some luck involved; initial research experiments seldom produce such dramatic results.

Still, in the end I believed I had proved my case. Now all I had to do was convince the rest of the medical community that I wasn't crazy.

You have to understand that doctors as a group are a pretty conservative bunch, professionally speaking. They know what they know what they know, and getting them to radically change what they're doing is a very tough sell.

So telling doctors that the resuscitation fluids they had been using on patients for decades were actually killing them was a glaring case of medical heresy. It was counter to everything they had learned and believed and practiced. Nevertheless, in addition to publishing my research results, I started going around to conferences and seminars, telling them that crystalloid solutions were harming their patients.

And the general reactions from surgeons and other trauma personnel were: 1) "Who is this Rhee guy?" and 2) "Whoever he is, he's nuts. I've given buckets of this stuff to patients for years, decades, and it doesn't do any harm." I didn't literally get booed off the stage, but it came pretty close.

Part of the problem was that I was still pretty young, in my late thirties, and I didn't yet have a national reputation. Fortunately, I soon acquired an important ally.

Dr. Ken Mattox was a nationally renowned cardiothoracic surgeon, a former protégé of famed heart surgeon Michael DeBakey, and chief of staff and surgery at Ben Taub General Hospital in Houston. Dr. Mattox was and is something of an iconoclast, not the sort of guy who was afraid to challenge current medical orthodoxy. During his lectures to other doctors he would sometimes show them a piece of medical equipment from three hundred years ago, a sort of bellowslike contraption that doctors of the time used to blow tobacco smoke into a patient's rectum. His point was that back then some of the greatest medical minds of the era actually thought that blowing smoke up a patient's ass was beneficial—so today's doctors shouldn't cling too strongly to the idea that the accepted medical practices of today are always the last word on the subject.

Anyway, Dr. Mattox had long been convinced that trauma surgeons and emergency medical personnel were giving trauma patients way too much resuscitative fluid. He proved his point by conducting one of the most difficult studies in medicine, demonstrating that trauma patients who didn't receive massive infusions of the crystalloid fluids had a higher survival rate than those who did. Fortunately for me, during his many visits to the USUHS medical school—he was an avid supporter of military medicine—it was my job as a junior surgeon to pick him up at the airport and drive him around. During one of these chauffeuring episodes I managed to get a word in and explained my research, which supported his opinion that fluids could be harmful. After that he started quoting me in his lectures, saying, "As Dr. Rhee demonstrated in the lab . . ." It gave me a lot more credibility.

Well, it was a long, hard road, but the eventual upshot of all this was that over the next decade it slowly came to be accepted that massive early infusion of crystalloid fluids in trauma patients was causing cellular damage and inflammation and death. I also helped demonstrate that hypertonic saline solution in the proper dose was a safe alternative to other fluids in treating blood loss, and that it was particularly beneficial with patients with penetrating traumatic brain injuries. It also has the added benefit of requiring just one eighth the volume and weight of lactated Ringer's solution—an important consideration for corpsmen, medics, and emergency personnel in the field.

Don't get me wrong. A lot of other people also worked on these issues, so no one person can take all the credit. But I hope that some of my work helped change the way we practice medicine.

And there is still plenty more to do in the field of resuscitative fluids. Earlier I said that during my lab experiments on the pigs I found that fresh whole blood was the very best resuscitative fluid—which may seem obvious. But whole blood is always in short supply, and storing it is difficult, so while it was routinely used in planned surgeries it was rarely used in trauma situations or on the battlefield, plasma or other blood products being the preferred alternatives. But as my experiments indicated, whole blood is so beneficial that it should be used whenever possible.

Which is why we set up a walking blood bank that time in Ramadi. Instead of giving the wounded troops clear fluids to get their blood pressure up, we'd replace the blood they had lost with blood that five minutes earlier had been coursing through a warm human body. And the results were almost miraculous. None of the wounded we treated with whole blood developed post-traumatic complications of the kind we had seen with other fluid resuscitations.

As for the supply and storage problems with whole blood, eventually those difficulties will be solved. I'm convinced that someday we'll be able to manufacture synthetic blood, where you'll have a machine on which you press a button and out comes a quart of O-positive or B-negative like cherry cola out of a slushy machine. It won't be easy, because blood is incredibly complex, with about a billion factors to it. In fact, I often say that whoever invented blood is a freakin' genius, and I'd really like to shake her hand. But someday it will happen.

There were other experiments I was involved with as well. I've already mentioned my work testing QuikClot, the hemostatic agent that I had used on the dying shooting victim at

County-USC. In those experiments, also with pigs, I was able to demonstrate that QuikClot was the most effective agent for stopping bleeding in areas that couldn't be accessed with tourniquets, such as groin wounds; the lab tests on QuikClot were a key factor in getting rapid FDA approval for its widespread and successful use by the Marines during the Iraq war. I also did research on the use of titanium staples instead of traditional sutures for quicker and easier repair of large vessels such as the thoracic aorta.

Another field of research in which I was involved was wireless vital-signs monitoring. When I was in Iraq I had always marveled at the high-tech wireless gear our soldiers had: computers, GPS, satellite imaging, personal communication devices, "blue force tracker" systems that allowed a commander to identify and pinpoint every tank and Humvee and truck in his command. Meanwhile, in my FRSS surgical unit at Ramadi it often seemed like we were working with two cans and a string. When we packed up patients for medevac, they'd be bristling with wires hooked up to bulky machines to monitor their vital signs during the flight. Once they were on the medevac choppers I had no way of knowing what was happening to them. I figured there had to be a better way.

So while I was in LA I wrote a grant request and got funds from the Office of Naval Research to develop a monitor that could wirelessly transmit data on a patient's blood pressure, pulse, and oxygen saturation to anyone with a receiver keyed into the system. Originally I approached NASA to develop a prototype, but while NASA is good at a lot of things, speed isn't always one of them. Frustrated by the bureaucracy, I finally found a small private company called Athena GTX to work on the project. What resulted was a device that weighed less than a pound and could be attached to a patient's blood pressure cuff at the scene of the injury. From that point it could transmit the patient's vital-signs data to a laptop or smart phone. After field testing by the military, including US Special Forces, Athena's Wireless Vital Signs Monitor was approved by the FDA for civilian use, and went on the civilian market at the beginning of 2011.

Of course, as a military man I didn't make any money off the invention. But as with my other research, I got something even more valuable—that is, the satisfaction of seeing my work help save lives in the field. As it turned out, one of the first civilian patients to benefit from the wireless monitoring device was Congresswoman Gabby Giffords. More on that later.

But perhaps the most potentially rewarding field of medical research I have been involved in concerns the use of "suspended animation" to treat severely injured trauma patients.

When I had first applied for the grant to study resuscitative fluids, the director of the Office of Naval Research program, Dr. Lynn Yaffe, said he'd give me the money on one condition—that I also look into suspended animation, the process of cooling down the human body and slowing the metabolic processes until the person is not quite dead but not exactly alive either. The heart stops beating, the lungs stop breathing, and, most important, brain cells and other cells being deprived of blood stop dying. The thinking was that if we could in effect "freeze" a mortally injured person, we would have a lot more time to repair the damage than we would if the patient were kept alive. Then, ideally, we could warm him back up and bring him back to life.

Well, at first this seemed way, way off the paved road, even for me. I mean, although therapeutic hypothermia had long been used in some medical procedures, everybody knew that hypothermia was fatal for trauma patients. We did everything possible to keep trauma patients warm, and now this guy was suggesting that we freeze them to death?

Still, I wanted the research grant, so I agreed. I started to get invited to "think tank" meetings where we would talk about how to do this and why. At one of them I met the late Dr. Peter Safar, the Austrian-born anesthesiologist who had invented CPR and who had done preliminary experiments on suspended animation. And the more I learned about suspended animation in humans, the more theoretically possible it seemed to be. What we needed to do was figure out the best way to do it.

For my experiments, Dr. Leon Sun, who was still working for me in the USUHS lab, and I took anesthetized man-sized pigs and surgically inflicted wounds to the aorta that caused them to start bleeding to death. Once their blood pressure dropped to near zero, we would infuse them with a cold (1 degree centigrade) solution containing potassium—the same substance used in lethal injections—to stop their heart and brain functions. Then we'd drain the rest of their blood, every drop of it, and replace it with a near-freezing fluid solution to cool the brain down to 10 degrees centigrade. With the animals now in a state of suspended animation—not quite dead, but not exactly alive—we could go in and at a leisurely pace repair the damage to the aorta. Then we would flush the cooling solution out of the pigs' venous systems and replace it with various rewarming solutions, including whole blood. And the pigs would come back to life.

Surgeons in the past had cooled patients down to about 18 degrees centigrade, which allowed them to stop circulation for about twenty to thirty minutes and then warm them up and bring them back. But the difference was that I had drained all the blood out of the pigs, filled them with a solution containing potassium at lethal doses, and then brought the animals back. Face it, when you are cold, with no blood or heartbeat, and full of potassium, you are definitely dead by anyone's definition.

I have to admit, the first time I saw a pig that had been clinically dead for a couple of hours suddenly rejoin the living, I could hardly believe it. It was as if, like Dr. Frankenstein, I had discovered the secret of life. None of my techs could believe it.

Again, this is all very simplified here. It wasn't a case of doing a few experiments on a few pigs and then running out and telling the world that the problem was solved. It took years, and dozens of individual experiments, to determine what cooling solutions were best, what temperatures were optimum, what worked and what didn't. Every question raised by skeptics—and there were many—had to be addressed.

For example, after publishing the results of early suspended-animation experiments, some people suggested that, sure, you could bring the pigs back to life, but they probably had suffered brain damage. I didn't think so, but I had to prove it—and how do you test a pig's learning and memory capabilities? It was pretty complicated, but basically I trained the pigs to recognize specially colored food boxes, and then tested them on it after they underwent the suspended-animation procedure. That experiment and others showed that the pigs could still recognize and remember the specially colored boxes, and thus that they had suffered no brain damage.

The potential implications of using suspended animation for severely injured trauma patients are enormous. As it is now, we have only twenty or thirty minutes to repair the damage to mortally injured trauma patients before they die, and often the extent of the injuries simply overwhelms the time we have to repair them. For a trauma surgeon, time is an implacable enemy. But what if we could stop the dying process in its tracks through hypothermic suspended animation? Then we'd have all the time in the world to fix the damage, and then bring the patient back to life. It could potentially save many, many lives. And maybe we wouldn't even have to wait until a trauma patient got to the hospital to start the process. What if medics or EMTs could induce suspended animation on the battlefield or at the scene of a shooting, halting the patient's dying process even before they got to the ER?

I know it sounds far-fetched. But if someone had told you fifty years ago that someday doctors would be able to take out a dead person's heart and stick it into someone else, or that they could put a laser on your eyeballs and you wouldn't need glasses, you'd have thought they were crazy. But now those things are routine.

It could be the same thing with suspended animation. What we have to do now is take it beyond pigs and into human clinical trials.

I worked on this for fifteen years before the Food and Drug Administration approved the suspended-animation process for human clinical trials with trauma patients in 2011. Dr. Samuel Tisherman, a longtime protégé of Dr. Peter Safar, had done many of the same kinds of experiments in their laboratory using dogs. Dr. Tisherman has been carrying on the ideas of Dr. Safar since his death and has been instrumental in going forward with this research into the human phase. With funding from the US Army, we'll do an initial feasibility study at the Shock Trauma Center in Baltimore, one of the busiest and best trauma centers in the country, and then the full trials will take place at five locations around the country, including at my shop at University Medical Center in Tucson. The trials will involve using my suspended-animation techniques only as a last resort for severely injured trauma patients who are demonstrably beyond the help of any conventional techniques—in other words, those who otherwise are surely going to die. I fully expect that the trials alone will save dozens of lives.

(Not everyone thinks this is such a great idea. After the FDA approval for clinical trials was announced, conspiracy theories about me and my work began circulating on the Internet. It's a little hard to follow, but apparently the theory is that in cooperation with the Pentagon I'm trying to use suspended animation to develop "zombie soldiers" as cannon fodder for the battlefield. I'm just guessing here, but I'm not sure the conspiracy theorists have fully reviewed the literature.)

Of course, completing the human clinical trials and transforming the theoretical to the practical will depend on getting sufficient funding—which I'll admit is kind of a sore point with me, not only in connection with my own research but with medical experimentation in general. I mean, we spend billions of dollars devising new ways to kill people; why can't we spend a billion or two to develop new ways to save people? Yes, I know that taxpayers often get annoyed when guys like me toss around numbers that start with a *b* like they were small things. But compared with the vast amounts we spend on other things, a billion really is chump change. I'm convinced that with a billion dollars, in ten years we could have this lifesaving procedure and technology on hand in every trauma center in America.

Well, as you can see, I get pretty passionate on the subject of medical research—as passionate as I am about being a trauma surgeon. That's why I spent so much time and effort on it, publishing more than two hundred peer-reviewed papers over the course of my career and giving over a thousand lectures and seminars. I think that the time I spent in the lab probably helped save more lives than I ever could have saved in an ER. For a medical researcher, seeing your work result in changes in medical procedure, seeing your work actually being put into play in the field, is the highest honor you can get, the greatest sense of satisfaction you can ever have.

And in fact four of the fields in which I had done lab research—resuscitation fluids and hypertonic saline, hemostatic agents, therapeutic cooling for trauma patients, and wireless vital-signs monitoring systems—would all play a role in helping people who were wounded on that bloody day in Tucson in January 2011.

CHAPTER 9

JANUARY 8, 2011

Things like this weren't supposed to happen in Tucson.

Most people in the greater Tucson area had always thought of their city as a safe place to live and raise a family, especially when compared with other metropolitan areas. The violent crime rate was relatively low, and most of that was concentrated in the central and southern parts of town. The suburban neighborhoods, like those near the La Toscana Village shopping center, were peaceful, quiet, orderly, safe, the kind of places where people weren't afraid to go jogging or walk their dogs at night. Certainly they weren't the kind of neighborhood where anyone would ever expect to be shot down in broad daylight by a stranger with a gun.

Sixteen seconds of gunfire on that Saturday morning in January 2011 shattered that illusion. It thrust the city of Tucson and the UMC Trauma Center, and trauma surgery in general, into the national spotlight.

That I was there when it happened was another one of those random twists of fate. In 2007, after twenty-four years of active service, I had been nearing the end of my Navy career and had to start looking for a job. I was still director of the Navy Trauma Training Center in Los Angeles, preparing Navy doctors and medical personnel for the harsh realities of war, and after six years the program was running smoothly. I loved the service and was grateful for the opportunities and adventures it had given me.

But it was time to go. I felt I had accomplished what I had wanted to do. And after so many transfers and stints of sea duty and overseas deployments I owed it to Emily and the kids to put down roots somewhere.

But where? My community of academic surgeons all knew I was retiring, and I had a lot of great offers. I was just about to accept an offer on the East Coast when at the last minute I was asked to look at a job as the chief of trauma at University Medical Center in Tucson. I knew that Tucson was somewhere in Arizona, but that was about it. But when I looked closer at the job, it met all the requirements. Tucson was big enough—metropolitan population just under one million—to support a Level I trauma center, and the university setting made it possible for me to remain an academic. I still wanted to do research and teach the next generation of young surgeons the things I had learned during two decades in the trauma business. But ironically, the most attractive thing about the UMC trauma program was that at the time there was hardly a trauma program at all. The program was in disarray, the funding was a major issue, and almost all the staff had left—which to me looked like an opportunity. I figured it couldn't get any worse, that the program had only one way to go, and that was up. Instead of stepping into an established program, I could build my own program and run it the way I thought a trauma program should be run. Building new programs was my specialty by now.

In short, it was a challenge. And I've always found it hard to pass up a challenge.

As it turned out, Tucson wasn't quite the bucolic, peaceful place that its boosters liked to think it was. In terms of traumatic mayhem it certainly wasn't equal to Los Angeles or Washington, DC, but it had its share. In an average year the UMC Trauma Center handles about five thousand trauma patients, everything from gunshot wounds to stabbings to car accidents to drownings and everything else. As chief of the trauma center with minimal help, I was back to working up to 120-hour weeks.

And building up the trauma program wasn't easy. There were endless bureaucratic struggles over money and resources and methods and practices, constant battles to make the trauma program the best it could be. When I got there, there was only one other trauma surgeon remaining in the program, Dr. Rifat Latifi, so he and I had to cover the trauma center by ourselves—which meant working thirty-six-hour shifts. Thirty-six hours of constantly running around with no sleep really takes a toll on your body. We had to have help, so when possible I would fly in a Navy surgeon moonlighting from Los Angeles, another surgeon from New York who used to live in Tucson, and a retired Navy surgeon from Phoenix. They provided enough relief until I was able to hire new surgeons.

But it was a struggle. When I was starting the new job, the advice that my colleagues gave me was, "Don't change anything for at least a year." I took this advice for about a week. The truth was, everything needed to be changed. I mean everything. And with so much to change, at first my style ruffled some feathers. Meanwhile, I was by myself, living in a tiny apartment while Emily and the kids were getting ready for the move from LA, working impossibly long hours, making the best of limited resources—in short, in a lot of ways it was like being on another overseas deployment, but much worse. That first year was one of the hardest times of my life.

The Arizona culture took a little getting used to as well. I remember when I first got to Tucson I went to a supermarket, one of those upscale supermarkets in the suburbs, and there was a middle-aged guy in jeans pushing a shopping cart with a Colt Peacemaker revolver in a quick-draw holster strapped to his leg. The dude was packing heat in a supermarket! That's not something you'd see in Washington, DC, or LA, but in Arizona it was perfectly legal, and not unusual. I remember thinking, Welcome to the Wild West.

But eventually everything worked out. Emily and the kids came out and we found a nice house outside the city. And after three years of hard work I had eight trauma surgeons in the program, backed up by a host of specialists—neurosurgeons, vascular surgeons, orthopedic surgeons—and a top-flight team of nurses and techs. As far as I was concerned, my trauma team was as good as any in the business.

That was why I didn't have to run faster when I got the call that Saturday morning that there were ten GSWs coming in. I knew the team in place that morning could handle things until I got there.

My work in the trauma center that morning began with a shout and a whistle—one of those long, loud, two-fingers-in-the-mouth whistles that is guaranteed to get everybody's attention.

"Eyes and ears on me, please!" I called out, and the various doctors and residents gathered around to give me a situation report. Again, we had been very lucky with the timing that morning. Dr. Randy Friese had been going off-shift and Dr. Narong Kulvatunyou had been coming on-shift when the shooting occurred, and Dr. Bellal Joseph was handling the surgical ICU, so we had three trauma surgeons available—four including me, although my primary job as chief of trauma was to command and control. When I'm on call I do all the required surgeries myself, and since this was a mass-casualty scenario I would do some surgery if it was necessary, if the other trauma surgeons were overwhelmed, or if there was some particularly tricky emergency surgery required. But mostly I was there to run the show. I had many hands that could do the work. What was really required of me was decision making and coordinating movements of patients and personnel.

My first job was to get a rundown on what we had.

In a trauma center the patients who come through the doors aren't initially identified by their actual names. Trauma victims often don't have ID on them, or even if they do, they may not be conscious and able to verify who they are. In other cases, such as gang shootings, we may want to keep their identities secret for security reasons. But especially in mass-casualty situations, or when we're having a busy day with a lot of patients, it's important that we're able to quickly distinguish each patient. So when they come in, we give each patient a "trauma name," a name that features a progressive two-letter code combined with a word chosen from an alphabetical list of randomly selected words. On this particular day the two-letter code was LB, and the alphabetical word list began with Ajo, Baja, Cactus, and so on. So the first patient's trauma name would be Ajo LB, the second Baja LB, the third Cactus LB, and on through the alphabet. It sounds a little confusing, but the system allowed trauma center personnel to immediately identify what day a patient came in and in what order.

Of course, later we would learn the actual names of the wounded who were being brought in. Later, too, we would learn about their families and the details of their lives, and exactly what had happened to them at the shooting scene.

But I didn't need to know that now, and in any event I didn't have time. Right now there were challenges that had to be met.

Randy told me that Baja LB—the trauma name for Congresswoman Giffords—had just been taken to the operating room. Dr. Martin Weinand was the neurosurgeon on call and was in charge of her care, but Randy wisely had also called in Dr. Michael Lemole, chief of neurosurgery at UMC, to assist. So we had two top-notch attending neurosurgeons there to operate on her. Dr. Kulvatunyou reported he had patients Cactus LB, Dune LB, Elk LB, and Falcon LB in trauma bays 3, 4, 5, and 6—more victims were still on the way—but they were under control. The scariest case he had was a middle-aged man, Globe LB, who had suffered gunshot wounds to the chest and leg. The leg wound was relatively minor, but Dr. K was afraid that Globe LB might have had injuries to his subclavian vessel, which was worrisome because these are huge veins and arteries under the collarbone that are extremely difficult to get to and control. This injury is a potential killer and one of the toughest to fix, so Dr. K wanted me to take this one on personally. (Later I would learn that Globe LB was Jim Tucker, a fifty-eight-year-old aerospace worker who had gone with his wife, Doris, to meet Congresswoman Giffords.)

Sure enough, Globe LB had a bullet hole and a large hematoma smack dab over the collarbone, which was obviously fractured from the bullet. Seeing that wound took me momentarily back to Ramadi, in Iraq, when we had a young soldier come in dead from a high-velocity gunshot wound that had blown out his collarbone and the subclavian artery. No blood pressure, no pulse; he had come to us dead. We had opened the young soldier's chest immediately, without even administering anesthesia as he was already clinically dead, and brought him back to life. We did this by putting a clamp on the subclavian artery as it came off the arch of the aorta through the chest to stop the bleeding from the severed artery that had been transected by the bullet. I then cut out his clavicle bone and performed a new trick that we were heavily promoting to the military surgeons training to go to the war: I inserted a six-inch "cannula," which is a little plastic tube about the size of a straw, into both cut ends of the vessel and tied them in place with sutures so the blood wouldn't leak out. It was a temporary shunt to link up both ends of the shattered vessel. The procedure not only controlled the bleeding but also allowed blood flow into his arm, which meant the arm wouldn't have to be amputated later. We packed him up and flew him out to Baghdad for the vascular guys to make permanent repairs. The young soldier lived.

Although I had been doing this shunting technique in civilian trauma for many years, and I had done it many times in Iraq, I was hoping I wouldn't have to do it now with Globe LB. But I was confident that if we needed to, we could do it again.

Globe LB's blood pressure was stable, meaning that it wasn't going down. We had put a large tube into his chest in the trauma bay to relieve the air and blood that had built up in the space between the lung and the chest wall, which could have killed him if not treated. The chest tube drains the blood and helps stop the bleeding, as well as letting the surgeons know how much blood the patient has lost and how much he may still be bleeding. It looked as though Globe LB may not have bled much, so that gave me time to get a CT scan to let me know what damage the bullet had caused internally. Eventually Globe LB would have to go to the OR to get his leg wound fixed, but that could wait until we could determine the extent of his other injuries. I ran off to the next trauma bay to check on Elk LB.

I later learned that Elk LB was Ron Barber, the congresswoman's district manager in Tucson. He had gunshot wounds in the thigh and the face. He was bleeding a lot from the leg wound, which could have indicated a femoral artery injury, but they had compression on it and it seemed to be under control. He and three other shooting victims that day had also benefited from the quick application of hemostatic bandages called Com-

bat Gauze by sheriff's deputies who had responded to the shooting scene—which was interesting. As noted earlier, I had done
extensive research on hemostatic agents in my lab, and had been
instrumental in getting QuikClot to the Marines when they went
to war in Iraq. Later the same company that made QuikClot,
Z-Medica, Inc., developed Combat Gauze, which was a field
dressing impregnated with the hemostatic product. When I first
arrived in Tucson, the sheriff's office had asked me if its deputies
should carry a hemostatic agent in the field, and if so, which one.
I had suggested Combat Gauze, and they had taken my advice.
For someone in academia, it's always professionally satisfying to
see your work pay off in the field.

It was Barber's other wounds that most worried me. He had
bullet holes in his cheek and mouth that went from front to back,
and the bullet had passed through his neck. Because of the trajectory, I was concerned that bullet might have hit his carotid
artery. On the other hand, he didn't look as if he had an expand-
ing hematoma, which is blood collecting under the skin. And
the neck on the side of the bullet track also didn't have a "thrill,"
which means that you can feel the blood passing under the swelling due to an injury in the artery. All that made a major arterial
wound seem less likely. I sent him off to the CT scanner to get a
better look at the bullet track.

The next patient, Falcon LB, had also been shot in the left
chest, right abdomen, and right leg; Dr. Joseph had already put a
chest tube in her. One look at her wounds told me what I needed
to know. I asked Dr. Joseph if he thought she needed to go to
the OR for an ex-lap, an exploratory laparotomy, an operation
in which we open up the abdomen to repair internal abdominal
injuries. He nodded, and I gave him the thumbs-up and said,
"Whenever you're ready." They started packing her up. Eventually I learned that she was Susan Hileman, fifty-eight, a neighbor

and friend of young Christina-Taylor Green. Only later would she be told that Christina-Taylor had died.

With three patients heading for the OR and one—Gabby Giffords—already there, I had to make sure everything was ready in the OR area, which was close to the trauma bays. As I ran over there, I was grateful that UMC wasn't like County-USC in LA, where fifteen flights of stairs had separated the trauma bay from the ORs. In the OR central desk area I checked the electronic board and saw that four of the fifteen ORs were in use for previously scheduled surgeries, and one, OR number 9, was currently occupied by Congresswoman Giffords. Once again, we were lucky that this was a Saturday, when far fewer surgeries were scheduled than on a weekday. If it had been a Monday, all of the ORs would have been in use except for one room that is always held in reserve for trauma cases. We were lucky, too, that one of the scheduled surgeries was being performed by Dr. Christy Smith. She was a crackerjack heart surgeon and would be able to help if I needed her. When I popped into her operating room she said, "I know, I know. I'm closing up right now and will be off the table right away. Do you need any help?" I told her I would, and to find me when she got finished.

I told the head charge nurse that I needed six ORs, fully prepped and staffed with anesthesiologists and OR nurses and techs. "Call in everybody," I said. At the time we had only four patients, including Giffords, who definitely needed surgery, but casualties were still coming in and I wanted to be certain we were prepared. Then I went into OR number 9, where Drs. Weinand and Lemole were getting Giffords ready for her surgery.

It was the first time I'd seen her. She had a wound on her forehead and a smaller wound in the back of her head. Her hair, which was matted with blood, was being shaved on the left side by Dr. Vern Fennell, a neurosurgical resident who was assisting Marty and Michael. A tube had been inserted into her throat to help her breathe and she was already on the anesthesia machine. After her hair was shaved away on her left side I looked at the hole in her forehead, then turned her head and examined the smaller hole in the back. Most of the skull damage was in the front, on the forehead over her left eye, which could have meant that it was the exit wound, that the bullet had entered the back of the head and exited at the front. Generally it's true that entry wounds are smaller than exit wounds, but it isn't always so—which is why in trauma we never label a wound as entry or exit but only by the location or number. The Giffords case was one of those exceptions. Later information from the shooting investigation, and a close examination of the CT scans, indicated that she had been shot in the front of the head, and that the smaller hole in the back was from a fragment of the bullet and not the entire bullet.

Once again, the fact that there were two holes was good news, because they sometimes reduce the pressure inside the skull from bleeding or swelling. I checked the monitors and saw that her blood pressure was a little low but stable, then looked at her CT scans, which were displayed on the monitors mounted on the wall of the OR.

"This looks pretty good. I'm very optimistic here," I told Marty and Michael, and we went over their operation plan while Vern placed the tongs in her skull, a kind of viselike device that holds the head perfectly rigid and in place.

"She's good to go," I said. I looked up at the anesthesiologists and asked if they needed anything and in a calm voice they responded, "No, Dr. Rhee, everything is fine and we have everything under control." I headed back to the trauma bay while Marty, Michael, and Vern started their incision and began their work.

I checked on Falcon LB, Susan Hileman, the woman with the chest wound, and got a thumbs-up from Dr. Joseph; she was packed up and ready to go to the OR. Ron Barber was still stable and waiting for his CT scan. I told Dr. K to be sure to get a good CTA—computed tomography angiogram, a technique that examines arteries and veins—of his neck, as he'd be next for surgery if needed. I checked the CT on Globe LB and saw that the subclavian artery looked okay, which was good news, but the bullet had damaged his lungs and he had air and blood in his chest. The chest tube we had inserted would help with that until we got him into surgery.

Meanwhile, Dune LB had a wound in the chest and his X-rays indicated blood in the chest, so I had a tube placed there to drain it and determine how much he was bleeding, and also to harvest any lost blood. As noted earlier, fresh blood has marvelous properties for postinjury recovery, and I always try to save as much clean thoracic blood from the patient as I can so I can infuse it back into the patient. Dune LB also was shot in the knee area and would need surgery for that, but not immediately. I needed to know if he was going to be stable and how much blood was coming out of the tube in the chest before I could decide when he would go to the operating room and for which procedure, the chest or the knee. Fortunately, an ultrasound done in the trauma bay showed that there hadn't been any injury to the heart.

Cactus LB was Pam Simon, Giffords's community outreach coordinator. She had been shot through the wrist, and then the bullet had grazed her right chest and entered her left chest. Oh, my God, I thought, another possible GSW to the heart. We assumed the bullet was in her chest, but bullets do strange things sometimes. After CT scanning her we finally discovered that this bullet had slung around under her skin and ended up near her left hip, fortunately without damaging any internal organs. We had planned to leave the bullet in there, which is the normal procedure if it isn't doing any more harm; taking it out is often medically riskier than leaving it in. But a lot of patients insist on having the bullets taken out. The thought of having a foreign body inside them is unsettling, and they worry about things like setting off metal detectors at the airport. A week later, after she'd been discharged, Pam asked to have the bullet taken out, as it was starting to get infected, and I did so. Pam likes to say that I took a bullet out of her butt, but that was only because of her incredible good luck. That bullet could have easily injured her heart and killed her.

Two other seriously injured patients who had originally gone to Northwest Medical Center, which was the closest hospital to the shooting scene but didn't have a trauma center, had also been rerouted to us. Hilo LB had been shot three times in the leg and was stable but would require surgery. She was Mavy Stoddard, seventy-five, whose husband, Dorwan, had been killed while he was trying to protect her from the gunman. Iron LB, a sixty-three-year-old man, had been shot in the knee and had another bullet that had shallowly penetrated the skin in his back; I eventually sent him up to the orthopedic OR to repair the broken knee. The orthopedic surgeons also took a bullet out of his side. Java LB came to the trauma center after initially being sent to St. Mary's Hospital. She was Mary Reed, fifty-two, who had been shot in the arms and back while protecting her seventeen-year-old daughter during the attack. She was stable, and I put her in line for a CT scan to determine the tracks of the wounds.

I found another patient, Kaibab LB, a sixty-year-old man, by himself in a regular ER room. He'd been shot in the ankle, but the bullet fortunately hadn't hit any major bones, and as part of the triage process he'd been directed to the ER instead of the trauma bay, which was filled with more seriously injured patients. He'd been bandaged, but everybody else was busy elsewhere and he was alone. I started to examine him, but he said to me, "Doc, I'm fine. Go take care of the others." He was a good guy. I found out later that he was Randy Gardner, a former mental health counselor, and that this was actually his second involvement in a mass shooting. As a young student at Kent State University in 1970, he had been in the crowd of anti–Vietnam War protesters when Ohio National Guard troops opened fire, killing four people.

(Three other patients with relatively minor wounds had been treated at Northwest Medical Center and released the same day. As later reported in the news, they were Bill Badger, seventy-four, a retired Army colonel who, despite being grazed on the head by a bullet, had been one of the people who helped subdue the shooter; Kenneth Dorushka, sixty-three, wounded in the arm and also treated and released; and Kenneth Veeder, seventy-five, an Army airborne veteran of Vietnam who was grazed in the leg.)

I also found one other patient very early on that day. As I passed by the elevators outside the trauma bay I saw two attendants with a gurney waiting for the elevator. On the gurney was a black plastic bag—what the military calls a body bag—and when I looked at it I saw that the form inside it was very small. I asked the attendants where they were taking this patient even though I already knew the answer. Although I didn't know her name yet, I knew this was the nine-year-old girl that Dr. Friese had tried to save but couldn't. In accordance with trauma protocols, she was being taken to the pediatrics ICU, where the staff was better prepared to deal with the dead bodies of children and the shattering grief of their parents.

I looked at that small form on the gurney for a moment, and then the elevator doors opened and she was taken away. I stood there for a few seconds, and then I had to tell myself to focus on the task at hand.

I kept on running. As I was heading back to the trauma bay, my cell phone rang again; it had been ringing all morning. My reaction was, What now? I checked the number and saw that it was a 202 area code—Washington, DC. I knew instantly who this call was going to be from. I answered and heard the familiar voice of Navy Commander Ronny Jackson, the White House assistant medical director.

I knew Ronny well. He'd been through my trauma training program at County-USC in Los Angeles, and we worked together in Iraq back in 2006.

"Captain Rhee," Ronny said, "POTUS [president of the United States] wants to know if you can give us any status on Congresswoman Giffords."

Still walking, I gave him a quick rundown on the congress-woman and the other casualties, ending with "Things are under control. She will do fine."

"If there's anything you need, we can get it for you," Ron said, and we hung up.

I wasn't surprised by the White House call. I knew that a mass shooting like this, especially in a usually quiet and safe sub-urban neighborhood, would garner some national news atten-tion. But I also knew the fact that a US congresswoman had been one of the people shot would turn an otherwise routine mass-shooting story—if a mass shooting can ever be called routine—into a major national event. No member of Congress had ever been shot down on the streets of America before. It was unprece-dented. So it was no surprise that the White House, and soon other powerful centers of government, would get involved.

I appreciated the offer of help if I needed it. As I said earlier, my philosophy is that everyone in my trauma center gets the best medical treatment I can provide, regardless of their position. And that rule still applied. But as a physician I wasn't about to turn down any special assistance to any of my patients if it was offered. If the White House or anyone else had resources that could help any of my patients, that was fine with me.

I also knew from personal experience that the White House had an almost unlimited ability to get things done. My first personal experience had occurred in 1998, when President Bill Clinton made a formal state visit to China. Ordinarily, when the president travels abroad the White House medical unit goes along in a plane equipped with an operating room staffed with a team of military doctors, nurses, and techs. But in this case the Chinese government had refused to allow the US medical plane to come into the country—probably because of questions of national pride. The Chinese government's attitude was that Chinese surgeons were perfectly capable of taking care of any emergencies. As you might expect, that was completely unacceptable to the Secret Service and the medical unit, especially after they had visited all the hospitals that would potentially be treating the president of the United States.

Eventually the two governments worked out a compromise. The president could bring his own trauma surgeon, but if anything happened he would have to operate on the president in a Chinese hospital. I got picked for the job. Traveling with President Clinton gave me an insight into things I had never thought of before and a much bigger picture of the world and how it works. And flying on Air Force One was awesome; you didn't even have to wear seat belts during takeoff or landing. Of course, nothing happened to the president during the trip, but I had to stay within steps of him, carrying a large pack of surgical instruments in case of an emergency. I was just one of the staff, invisible to the press cameras, but I got a firsthand presidential tour of China, from Tiananmen Square to the Great Wall. And after seeing the White House staff in action, I knew they could make things happen that otherwise wouldn't be possible.

Anyway, after Ronny's call I ran back to the trauma bay and gave another whistle and shout—"Eyes and ears on me!"—and a doctor or resident assigned to each of the cases gathered around to give me an update. People started shouting out reports: Globe LB's CT scan showed that the bullet did not hit the subclavian artery. Ron Barber's CT scan showed no carotid artery injury; the bullet had missed it by a few millimeters. He had a fracture to his mandible, and he would still need to go to the operating room soon to fix the injuries in his leg. I looked at Dr. K and gave him the green light to get him into the OR to work on the bleeding gunshot wound in the thigh. Falcon LB, Susan Hileman, was now in the OR for an ex-lap. Iron LB was in the OR with the orthopedic surgeons. All the other patients were stable and under control, but I was updated on every injury they had. I still had to get Cactus LB, Pam Simon, and others to the OR, but we had time.

Next I jogged over to the command center next to the trauma bay, where the hospital administrative director, chief medical officer, nursing director, public information officer, and others were waiting for an update. I gave them a complete list of the injured—except for Congresswoman Giffords, all of the injured had been able to speak and confirm their actual names—and made certain all the security measures were in effect. I told them to start getting together the injured patients' family members who were waiting outside. Then I headed back to the OR.

I checked on Congresswoman Giffords and found that Marty and Michael were about an hour into what would be a two-hour surgery. The surgery we had decided on for her was somewhat controversial, a procedure known as decompressive craniectomy—that is, relieving pressure on the swollen brain by removing portions of the skull.

The usual procedure is to drain the bleeding blood clot around the brain to allow more room for the brain to expand inside the skull and relieve some of the pressure, and then to put the removed portion of the skull back on. But this only works if the swelling is minimal. If the swelling is severe and you put the skull back on, the pressure can really build up. This not only restricts blood flow to the brain, but it gets so tight inside the skull that the brain herniates, meaning it gets squished through the opening at the base of the skull where the spinal cord comes out. Herniation is fatal to the brain. You become brain-dead. Your body may remain alive, but your mind and soul are gone. A decompressive craniectomy will prevent herniation by opening up the skull for brain expansion, but there are downsides to that, too. As an unrestrained brain swells it stretches, and that isn't good because, to put it simply, brain cells aren't stretchy. The potential effects on long-term recovery aren't yet fully known.

So it's a case of choosing the lesser of two evils. In Congresswoman Giffords's case, however, the bullet partly made the decision for us. The bullet had already performed a partial craniectomy, as the skull was fractured and the pressure was already relieved, so we decided it was best to surgically remove portions of the left side of her skull and preserve them in case they were needed later when the skull was reconstructed. (These days a composite material is generally used for skull reconstruction instead of natural bone, but it's best to keep the skull fragments anyway, just in case.) We decided not to try to remove any bone fragments or bullet shards deep in the brain that were not easily within reach, as that could pose more danger than leaving them in place. All in all, her brain looked relatively good; it wasn't pulsating, which is often a sign of severe inflammation.

Michael gave me a thumbs-up on Giffords, which meant that all was going according to plan. I checked in with the anesthesiologists, and they were happy at their end. It was great news. Although I couldn't know what Giffords's long-term prognosis was—to what extent she would be able to recover her functions—at this point I already knew this much with certainty: she was not going to die.

I checked on Falcon LB, Susan Hileman, who was undergoing the ex-lap, and Dr. Joseph told me it looked like she was okay, that there was no damage to any major organs or arteries. Dr. K, who was with Ron Barber, had clamped off a femoral vein and was turning the case over to Dr. John Hughes, a highly experienced vascular surgeon who had been called in and who ultimately did a venous repair. I remember worrying about the nerve next to the vessels. I saw the injuries and knew that the bullet path might leave him with a permanent deficit. I hoped he would recover. I then checked the orthopedic OR where Iron LB was getting his fractured knee washed out. I asked the orthopedic surgeon, Dr. Michael Miller, if he could also remove the bullet in his back, which was just below the skin. He said no problem. That bullet and the bullets from all the other patients retrieved by us would later be turned over to the FBI for analysis and identification.

On my way back to the trauma bay I ran into Dr. Christy Smith, the cardiothoracic surgeon who had been performing a scheduled surgery when the trauma victims came in. She offered to take a look at the CT scan on Globe LB, the man with the possible subclavian artery damage. After looking it over, she said it looked like everything was okay to her, that the artery was fine and the patient wouldn't need any further work.

Once again it struck me how lucky we had been with this mass-casualty situation. In addition to having had four trauma surgeons (me included) at the trauma center, we'd had a cardiothoracic surgeon on-site and two neurosurgeons, a vascular surgeon, and an orthopedic surgeon within easy reach. I could hardly have asked for a better supply of resources. It sounds odd to say it, but compared with other mass-casualty situations I'd handled, especially in Iraq, this was a piece of cake, a trauma director's dream come true.

Two hours after the first patient came in, everything was under control. All of the patients were stable or in the OR. None of them was going to die. Now it was time to tell their family members so.

About thirty people were gathered in a section of a large meeting room, waiting for news; other family members hadn't arrived yet. The hospital had a team of counselors standing by to help. When I walked in, a list of the injured in hand, the family members all looked at me with the same fearful expressions I had seen so many times before.

I called out the names of each patient, and when the family members came forward we went into a separate smaller room, where I gave them a quick rundown on their loved one's injuries and condition. In each case I was able to assure them that even if the injuries were serious, their loved ones were not going to die. I didn't have time to do much other than give them the bare facts, but it was pretty much all good news, medically speaking. The sad part was that most of the wounded patients had family members or friends who were among the dead.

After briefing the patients' family members, I went back to the OR to check on progress. Marty and Michael had finished with the congresswoman, who would soon be on the way to the ICU. The other OR patients' surgeries were all nearly completed as well. I took another quick run down to the trauma bay, where everyone seemed to be doing well. The surgical ICU was quickly making room for the onslaught of patients that were about to come out of the OR, the wards were all making room and the maintenance crew was busy cleaning rooms. Everyone was there, and the machinery was all humming at high speed.

Now, a little over three hours after the first patient had arrived, I had to meet the press.

At the earlier meeting at the command center I had stressed to the hospital administration how important it was that the reporters who were flocking by the dozens to the hospital be given as much information as possible. Information is the news media's lifeblood, and if we didn't give it to them they would simply try to get it elsewhere—and if that happened, chances were the information would be wrong. There already had been an erroneous news report that the congresswoman had died, a report that had spread like wildfire from one news organization to the other before it was finally discounted. I wanted to make sure the press, and thus the public, got the story straight. And since I was the only person who had an overall view of all the patients and injuries involved, I decided I should be the source of that information. Everyone agreed.

It wasn't that I craved the limelight. In fact, I still hadn't completely gotten over my youthful shyness and fear of speaking to large groups. But I had dealt with the press before, especially in Los Angeles, where there had been a lot of stories written and broadcast about the Navy Trauma Training Center. I felt like I could handle the situation. Although I had never had formal media training, I was used to speaking to large audiences when presenting my research papers.

Even so, I wasn't quite prepared for the scale of press interest in the case, that day and in the days that followed. At two P.M., I walked out to the podium in a large hospital conference room in front of about sixty reporters and TV camera crews, most of them from Tucson and Phoenix network affiliates; the national reporters were still on the way. I was still wearing scrubs and a brown-yellow-and-green-camouflage surgical cap. It may have looked a little odd to the TV viewers, who probably expected to see someone in a suit, or maybe a white lab coat. But I was still working, so I was wearing my working clothes.

I gave a quick one-minute statement—ten patients received, one dead at the hospital, five in critical condition and in the OR, all the others stable with no life- or limb-threatening injuries. The first question from the press was, "Is the congresswoman deceased?"

"No, the congresswoman is not deceased," I said. "She is in critical condition, but at the current time I'm very optimistic about recovery."

"Where was she shot?" a reporter asked.

"In the head," I said. I went on to explain that she had been shot once, through and through, and that the bullet had gone through her brain. I said that we couldn't be sure about the extent of her recovery, but I added, "I'm about as optimistic as I can get in this kind of situation."

My answers seemed to surprise the reporters—and probably many TV news viewers as well. How could someone be shot through the brain and still be alive, much less have a surgeon "optimistic" about her recovery? I didn't have the time or the inclination to explain to them in detail about why I was optimistic—the track of the bullet, Giffords's ability to follow commands, and other factors. They would just have to take my word for it.

There was one moment in the press briefing that surprised me. After I had said that the congresswoman was not dead, a reporter naturally asked me who had died. I couldn't give them a name, but I said, "I can tell you that the person who died here at the hospital was a young child."

The moment I said that, there was an audible gasp from the

crowd of reporters, and several shocked cries of "Oh, my God!" It wasn't what I expected from a crowd that was used to covering other people's tragedies. But maybe I shouldn't have been surprised. Reporters are people, too.

The press briefing lasted only a few minutes. I went back to the trauma bay and the OR area. Everything was under control. Then I went to the ICU, where the congresswoman was coming out from anesthesia.

I wanted to keep her in a medically induced coma, which limits the electrical activity in the brain and helps the damaged brain tissue to heal. To do that I put her on a propofol and fentanyl drip, which are ultra-fast-acting drugs. (Yes, propofol is the same drug that was misused so badly in the death of Michael Jackson.) The advantage of these types of drugs is that not only are they ultra-fast-acting, they're also ultra-fast-stopping; as soon as you turn off the drip, their effects disappear and you can measure the brain's functionality.

Unfortunately, when people heard that Giffords was in a medically induced coma, they ignored the "medically induced" part and concluded that Giffords was in a coma, which they assumed could last for months or years. The truth was that we could bring her in and out of a comatose state at will. A very short time after she came up to the ICU, when things were stable and calm, I stopped the drugs: I wanted to see how she was and I wanted her to wake up. Within half an hour, she started to move spontaneously, and when I asked her to show me two fingers she lifted up the first and second fingers on her left hand. That told me what I had already believed to be true: she was going to survive. I turned the drugs back on to give her a rest until the next day.

I also infused the congresswoman with a 5 percent hypertonic saline solution, the same solution I had conducted so many research experiments on when I was in Washington, DC. Its use had remained controversial—as noted earlier, the medical establishment is notoriously slow to adapt to new techniques—but I had been using it on brain trauma patients for years and its effects are really beneficial. I had to fight when I first got to Tucson to use this fluid, but now it had become routine. It helps reduce the swelling in the brain in many ways, but one of the main ones is that it lets me increase blood volume in the body without the deleterious effects that normal IV fluids can have. As I discovered in my research, it also helps cell immunology. I was convinced it would improve Giffords's chances for long-term recovery.

By this time Congresswoman Giffords's husband, Mark Kelly, had arrived at the hospital. He'd been in Houston, where he was training his team as the commander of the next scheduled Space Shuttle flight, when one of Giffords's staff members called him with the awful news. A corporate executive friend of his had given him the use of his private plane, and Mark and his two children and his mother had flown to Tucson. During the flight he and his family members had heard the news reports that Giffords was dead, and although he quickly determined that the reports were false, it had been a terrible shock.

At the hospital Mark was joined by Giffords's parents, Spencer and Gloria Giffords, who lived in Tucson. Randy, Marty, Michael, and I took Mark into a room and explained the situation to him, going over the congresswoman's injuries and the treatment she had received so far. Mark was clearly under enormous emotional distress, but at the same time he was calm and completely under control. That wasn't surprising to me. Navy captains, much less astronauts, are not by nature given to panic.

The information we could give him was reassuring, but also conditional. Yes, I told him, your wife is going to survive. I was absolutely certain of that. But, no, we can't say for certain what the length and extent of her recovery will be. Only time will tell.

Mark asked the right questions and calmly took in the answers. As soon as possible he was allowed to go into the congresswoman's room in the ICU, where he sat by her bedside, surrounded by a constant stream of doctors and ICU nurses. Throughout the night and into the next day, whenever I checked on Giffords, which was often, he was still sitting there, wide awake, gently holding her hand.

All through the day I had been so busy inside the hospital that I hadn't been aware of what was happening outside the hospital. But when I made a quick stop at my office I looked out the window and saw that hundreds of people had gathered in front of UMC, standing in silent vigil for the injured. They had also constructed a kind of impromptu memorial on the front lawn, filling it with candles and photographs and crosses and flowers. The vast majority of them hadn't personally known Congresswoman Giffords or Christina-Taylor Green or any of the other victims, but they somehow felt a need to be there, to express with their presence their grief for the dead and their hopes for the injured.

This was something new to me. In my many years of dealing with victims and their families, I had seen no small share of grief and anguish—patients screaming in the trauma bay, families crying in a waiting room, tough young Marines and soldiers weeping as their comrades lay wounded in a forward surgical unit. But I had never personally seen a mass expression of grief like this.

And it wasn't just in Tucson. All day long I had been getting phone messages and e-mails from across the country, from friends, military and medical colleagues, and high-level government officials offering help, including the head of the congressional medical unit and several NASA officials. Although I hadn't had a chance to watch the news, it was clear that the nation was watching what was happening in Tucson.

But of course the world hadn't stopped turning, and the doors to the trauma center hadn't stopped swinging. In the hours just after the Giffords shooting we had five more patients come in. One was an elderly man who had fallen down and hit his head, a problem compounded by the fact that he was taking anticoagulants; he kept the neurosurgeons working all night to stop the bleeding in his brain. Just after midnight another patient came in, shot in the heart. We opened him up as soon as he got inside the trauma bay, but the bullet had also hit the large vessels in his abdomen, and he died.

And on and on. I kept making the endless rounds—trauma bay to OR to ICU and back again—working on the new patients and checking on the old ones. I called Emily to give her an update and to tell her, as I had so many times before, that I wouldn't be coming home that night. At three A.M., after being up for more hours than I could remember and attending to more than two dozen seriously injured patients, I finally lay down on a couch for a few hours' sleep.

Like I said. Another day at the office.

CHAPTER 10

AFTERMATH

For the slain victims of the Tucson shootings, the gunfire that erupted on the morning of January 8, 2011, was an ending, the end of lives cut short for no reason. But for the wounded survivors of those brief moments of terror, the shootings at the Tucson shopping center were a beginning—the beginning of weeks, months, even years of recovery not only from their physical wounds but from psychological ones as well. From long experience with the victims of violent trauma I knew that even after their bodies healed, their lives would never quite be the same.

I woke up Sunday morning after a few hours of fitful sleep on my office couch and immediately headed for the ICU. Six of the mass-shooting patients were there, all resting as comfortably as could be expected, none showing any signs of postoperative complications. Some would be discharged in a day or two, while others would require further surgeries. Still, with so many bullets hitting so many human bodies it was something of a miracle that so few of the survivors had suffered damage to major organs or arteries.

Congresswoman Giffords was of course the exception. By far the most seriously wounded of the group, it was still too early to tell what her long-term prognosis would be. But there continued to be encouraging signs. If she remained in her present condition, it boded well for her recovery; if she started to backslide, if the brain swelling increased, more surgery might be required.

I was confident that Giffords was receiving the very best treatment and care that American medicine had to offer. But Mark Kelly and I agreed that it might be useful to get a second opinion from some nationally recognized doctors, not only to validate what we were doing but also to document what we were doing from a historical point of view. I knew this case would long be studied as an example of state-of-the-art trauma surgery at this time. And since I had the full support of the White House and Congress, I knew I could get the guys I wanted for the job—Jim Ecklund and Geoff Ling. They were both eager to help.

Col. Geoff Ling was vice chairman of the neurology department and director of the Division of Critical Care Medicine at the Uniformed Services University of the Health Sciences in Bethesda, Maryland, my alma mater, and a longtime friend. He was probably the world's best and most renowned neurointensivist—that is, a specialist in brain resuscitation. Jim Ecklund was a retired Army colonel who previously had been chief of neurosurgery at Walter Reed Medical Center before going into private practice. A West Point graduate, he had been the US Army's top brain surgeon and was a classmate of mine from medical school. They both had extensive experience in treating penetrative brain injuries in military personnel from the wars in Iraq and Afghanistan.

In fact, when I called Geoff at home that Sunday morning I learned he was getting ready to leave the very next day for another trip to Afghanistan. He was at the store picking up some last-minute stuff for his deployment when I called, but his wife told me, "He's going to be really sorry that he won't be able to come out to Tucson, Peter." But a few phone calls later, Geoff got pulled off his plane to Afghanistan by order of the office of the Joint Chiefs of Staff and headed out to Tucson.

When Geoff and Jim arrived and went over everything we had been doing, they were happy with what they saw. I had been a little concerned that they might question my use of hypertonic saline to raise the congresswoman's sodium level, which absorbs water and reduces brain swelling; as I said, it was still a somewhat controversial treatment. I had actually raised her sodium level to a little less than I might otherwise have because I didn't want it to seem like I was running any unproven treatments on her. The funny thing was, when Geoff looked at all the data, he told me, "Peter, you've done everything exactly right—except I would have given her *more* hypertonic saline."

After they looked things over, both Geoff and Jim concluded that the treatment had been exactly what they would have done themselves. They both assured Mark Kelly that his wife was getting the best possible care, which made him feel better—and made me feel better, too.

Meanwhile, press and public interest in the congresswoman and the other victims was only getting bigger.

Outside the hospital that Sunday morning, people by the hundreds were still coming by to add to the impromptu memorial on the front lawn, piling it high with get-well letters and flowers and candles; one veteran even left the Purple Heart he had received when he was wounded in Iraq. Thousands of other calls and letters were coming in from across the nation and around the world, expressing condolences and hopes for the victims. Again, every mass shooting in America garners a lot of press and public attention, but this was different somehow. Certainly the fact that a congresswoman had been shot, and in the public view was desperately clinging to life, added to the drama. But whatever the reason, I had never seen anything like it.

The crowds of reporters were also growing, not only from the national newspapers and networks but from international news organizations as well: Telemundo, the BBC, Al Jazeera, and on and on. In keeping with my policy of giving press members the information they needed so they wouldn't get incorrect information elsewhere, Dr. Michael Lemole and I gave daily press briefings, and I made myself available when possible for individual interviews with the major news networks.

Perhaps as was to be expected, they all wanted to know about the congresswoman, to the point where, frankly, I started getting a little annoyed. I occasionally had to remind the reporters that there were other victims of the shooting as well, and in the press briefings over the next days I sometimes introduced family members of the other victims to make sure they weren't forgotten.

As for discussing the congresswoman's injuries and prognosis, I wanted to be as direct and open as I could be. At first Mark Kelly was leery of this approach. He was still understandably upset about the initial reports that the congresswoman had died, and was worried that the news media would twist or sensationalize the information if it were released. But after hearing from friends about some of the early news coverage, much of which was wrong, he realized it was better to tell the press and public what they wanted to know.

"Peter, you're right," he told me. "Give them the information they want. There is a lot of misinformation out there."

So with Mark's permission and permission from the other victims and their family members, I tried to be as informative as I could be. I also kept expressing my continued firm belief about the congresswoman's survival, and my growing optimism that she would experience some significant recovery. But I could tell from the reporters' questions that they still weren't quite buying it, that they still couldn't quite believe that someone with a bullet through the brain could actually survive. Finally I decided to be even more emphatic. When a reporter asked me again about her chances of survival, I responded, "She has a 101 percent chance of surviving. She will not die."

The "101 percent chance" remark made headlines around the country. And for the first time, I think, people started to believe it.

Not everyone approved of the remark. Some of my medical colleagues and members of the public thought the "101 percent" statement sounded overconfident, even cocky, that there was no way I could make such a promise. But unlike the critics, I had spent my life dealing with traumatic injuries, including brain injuries like the one Giffords had suffered, and everything I knew, everything I had experienced with countless other patients, indicated that she would live. It was what I believed, and so it was what I said.

The "101 percent" statement also had a curious side effect. Because I was so certain of her survival, there was some speculation in the news media on the injuries that she sustained. Some people actually thought that she must have suffered only a minor injury, a glancing blow, and that she and we had merely been lucky. Otherwise how could she still be alive? Well, she certainly had been lucky in many ways, but she had suffered a devastating through-and-through gunshot wound to the brain. And I'm convinced it was only through the efforts of our trauma team that she had survived.

Her survival was not a fluke. When I first came to Tucson in 2007 to build the UMC trauma program, the survival rate for people with gunshot wounds in the brain was 10 percent—about the national average. Many victims of gunshot wounds to the brain were being allowed to die because the chances of survival and the recovery of physical and mental capacities were so low. But through a program of aggressive treatment by our trauma team, including emergency brain surgery, within a year the survival rate had increased to 24 percent, then 35 percent. By 2011, the year the congresswoman was shot, the survival rate for patients with gunshot wounds to the brain who were treated by our trauma team stood at 46 percent. In 2011, we treated twenty-eight patients with gunshot wounds to the brain, including the congresswoman, and thirteen of them survived. True, most of them faced extensive rehabilitation, and others were left in vegetative states and eventually would be removed from life support. But the point is that because of our trauma team's efforts, they had a chance at life that they otherwise would not have had.

Some question the need for having trauma systems in place, as they can be expensive. But I think our numbers speak for themselves.

In any event, I think the open policy with the press worked. From what I saw, after that first hectic day there was almost no incorrect medical information about the shooting victims in the news. I think the policy benefited University Medical Center and the trauma program as well. The press coverage of the hospital and its staff was nothing short of glowing. I never heard one suggestion that Congresswoman Giffords or any of the other victims would have been better off somewhere else.

The openness with the press, and thus the public, also put a positive face on trauma surgeons in general. Instead of looking guarded and uncertain, every one of the doctors who was interviewed by reporters—Dr. Friese, Dr. Joseph, Dr. Lemole, me—came off looking confident, decisive, thoroughly knowledgeable: all the qualities that you want in a surgeon, and especially a trauma surgeon. I was proud of my hospital, of my colleagues, of my profession, and I wanted to get that message out to the public.

And as it turned out, I would soon have an opportunity to get that message across to the most powerful person in America.

Shortly after the Tucson shooting, plans were announced for a memorial service to be held for the victims on Wednesday, January 12. It was soon announced that President Barack Obama and First Lady Michelle Obama would attend the memorial service, along with a host of other high-ranking government officials.

I wanted the president to come to the hospital as well, not just to visit Congresswoman Giffords and the other shooting victims but also to get a firsthand look at the trauma center and to meet the trauma team members. I thought it would be good for the hospital, good for the trauma program, and good for the team. And what better way to get the message out about the importance of trauma medicine than to show it to the president of the United States?

My friend Cmdr. Ronny Jackson of the White House medical unit had come out to Tucson, so I mentioned it to him and he took it up with the White House staff. Based on my earlier experience with President Clinton's trip to China, I knew the White House staff and the Secret Service would want a minute-by-minute plan for the visit. Instead of waiting for them to come up with one, I drew up my own: "3:10 P.M., POTUS enters building; 3:12 P.M., POTUS enters ICU; 3:13 P.M., POTUS goes to Giffords's room," and so on. When the president's advance team showed up to check things out, I gave them the proposed schedule and they approved it start to finish.

The president and the first lady arrived at the hospital at about 3:30 P.M. that Wednesday. Michelle Obama, surrounded by staff and Secret Service agents, came into the ICU first, where I and other trauma and surgical critical-care staff members were waiting. I had made sure that everyone who'd been involved in treating the shooting victims was there.

Mrs. Obama was incredibly gracious, thanking all of us for what we had done. Then, right behind her, President Obama came in.

I don't know if it's the aura of the office or the quality of the man—maybe it's both—but when the president of the United States walks into a room, the atmosphere instantly changes. The room falls silent, every eye focused like a laser beam on one person: the president.

I introduced myself and then led the president and first lady to Congresswoman Giffords's room, where Mark Kelly and her parents were waiting. Before we went in, I briefed them both on the congresswoman's condition and progress. I also prepared them for her physical appearance, which is something you often have to do with friends and family members of trauma victims; in a lot of cases the patients look worse than they actually are. In Giffords's case, she was still on a breathing tube, her head had been shaved on the left side, and she was heavily bandaged on her right eye, the eye socket having been damaged by the bullet. But I told them to feel free to ask her questions, and to assume that she could hear and understand what they were saying to her. Inside the room they greeted Mark and the congresswoman's parents and then the president and first lady stood by her bed, holding her hand. The president told her that he was proud of her, and that the entire nation was praying for her.

The president and the first lady stayed with Mark and Gabby for a while, then I led them to the rooms of four other victims of the shooting, including Ron Barber and Pam Simon. Along the way I introduced him to every doctor, resident, and nurse I could. President Obama has that politician's gift of being able to make everybody he meets feel like they're the most important person in the world. He thanked each of them, praised the work they had done, said the country was proud of them, and made a point of having the White House photographer in the entourage get a photo together with each one of them. They of course were awestruck. What was amazing to me was that I introduced him to dozens of people, and when he passed by them later in the tour he called them by name.

Although I was busy leading the president on his tour and didn't see it, something else happened during the presidential visit that was noteworthy. Moments after the president left the congresswoman's ICU room, two of Giffords's friends from Congress, Senator Kirsten Gillibrand and Representative Debbie Wasserman Schultz, came to her room for a visit, along with House minority leader and former speaker Rep. Nancy Pelosi. As they stood next to Giffords's bed, talking to her, Giffords's left eye started to open. Mark rushed to her bedside and called out, "Open your eyes, Gabby!" She did, and Mark said, "Honey, if you can see me, put your thumb up." She lifted her left arm and raised her thumb. Later everybody who was there, as well as the news media, called it a miracle.

Well, there were a lot of miracles associated with Gabby Giffords's survival and recovery, and maybe opening her eye when she did was one of them; certainly it was a good sign of continuing recovery. But medically, it was a predictable miracle. As noted, I had been using propofol and fentanyl to put the congresswoman on a sleeping and waking schedule—sleeping in a comalike state so her brain could heal, then waking so her functionality could be assessed. Over the past few days she had been able to hear and follow commands—show me two fingers, et cetera—and her left eye had flickered slightly open on command. Based on my experience with other traumatic brain-injury patients, I had expected her to spontaneously open her eye during her waking period that day—which, as it turned out, coincided with the exact time of the visit from the president and the congresspeople. That morning, in fact, at a meeting with the hospital administrative staff I had predicted that the congresswoman would open her eye during the president's visit—and while some of the staff had doubted the prediction, I hadn't been off by much.

Still, I didn't tell anybody that at the time. As Dr. Michael Lemole told a reporter who asked about the eye opening, "We would be wise to acknowledge miracles." And he was right.

After the president's visit, he and the first lady left by motorcade to the university's McKale Memorial Center arena for the memorial service. I had been invited to attend to represent the medical center, so I rode along in another limo in the motorcade. I was still wearing scrubs and a white lab coat. Later, during a reception following the memorial service, President Obama asked me why I was still wearing scrubs. I told him, "Because you're here."

You see, whenever the president travels, the chief of trauma in that city is put on alert in case anything happens to him—and in this case, that was me. When the president is in the city, I am on call in case he gets shot or injured. It's the same in all cities. The White House medical unit has a contingency plan on what exactly to do at all times if the president is injured. They even have the exact routes planned to get him to the trauma center from every place he goes, right down to every turn his limo will take while in transit.

The arena was packed to capacity with fourteen thousand people and another thirteen thousand in overflow watching on a Jumbotron at the football stadium; it seemed like all of Tucson had turned out for the event. I was supposed to meet Emily and the kids there, but I couldn't find them, so I went running through the crowds looking for them.

And then a strange thing happened. I started hearing people cheering and clapping, and at first I thought some celebrity must be coming through the crowd. But when I looked around I realized they had recognized me from the TV briefings and interviews, and they were cheering for me. Over the years I'd had countless patients and family members thank me for helping them, but no crowd of people had ever cheered me before. It was a very strange feeling. My attitude then and since is that the cheering wasn't for me personally, but for my trauma team. Still, it was very gratifying to see the expressions on my wife's and kids' faces when they saw their dad being treated like he was some kind of a hero. They were so used to what I do that they never saw me in this way.

The arena was full of high-level government officials, as well as with many of the first responders and families of the victims. There were remarks from Homeland Security secretary Janet Napolitano, Arizona governor Jan Brewer, Attorney General Eric Holder, and Daniel Hernandez Jr., an intern in Giffords's office who had rushed to her side after the shooting. Then the president went to the podium.

I thought it was one of the best speeches President Obama ever gave. He called for unity and civility in the face of tragedy, and gave tributes to each of the dead: Judge John Roll, a University of Arizona law school graduate who had served our legal system for nearly forty years; Dorothy "Dot" Morris, who died despite the efforts of her high school sweetheart and husband of fifty years to protect her; Phyllis Schneck, mother of three, grandmother of seven and great-grandmother of a two-year-old girl; Dorwan Stoddard, who died trying to protect his wife, Mavy; Gabe Zimmerman, Gabby Giffords's outreach director, who had devoted himself to serving constituents in need; and nine-year-old Christina-Taylor Green, a dancer, a gymnast, a swimmer, the only girl on her Little League team, a young girl who embodied the hopes for the future.

It was all incredibly moving. But the part of his speech that struck me most was this: "Sudden loss causes us to look backward," the president said, "but it also forces us to look forward; to reflect on the present and the future, on the manner in which we live our lives and nurture our relationships with those who are still with us. We may ask ourselves if we've shown enough kindness and generosity and compassion to the people in our lives. Perhaps we question whether we're doing right by our children, or our community, whether our priorities are in order. We recognize our own mortality, and we are reminded that in the fleeting time we have on this Earth, what matters is not wealth, or status, or power, or fame, but rather, how well we have loved and what small part we have played in making the lives of other people better."

During my career I had seen countless cases of lives suddenly lost, had seen the pain of loss etched on countless faces of family members and friends. I had always wondered if in the midst of seemingly senseless tragedies there was anything positive to be gained, any lesson to be learned. The president said the answer was yes. However sudden and tragic, death calls upon us to be kind and loving to the living.

The memorial service and the president's address were an emotional catharsis for Tucson and for the nation. The TV news crews remained, and Michael and I continued to give our daily briefings. But slowly things began to return to normal.

Actually, for those of us at the UMC Trauma Center, things had never stopped being normal, in the sense that patients had continued to stream in through the doors. On the Sunday after the mass shooting we had thirteen cases come in: two guys who had tried and nearly succeeded in beating each other to death in a drunken family brawl, five car accidents, a motorcycle rider run over by a car, a bicycle rider clipped by an SUV, a guy who broke his back when he flipped his all-terrain vehicle, and—only in Tucson—three people with broken bones after falling off horses. The flow of patients never stopped.

Except for Gabby Giffords, all of the wounded from the shooting were discharged within a week, some of them to begin a long period of rehabilitation. Congresswoman Giffords continued to improve. I wanted to start stimulating her brain right away, and getting her up and moving was the best way to do that. Kara Snyder, one of the best critical-care nurses I have ever met, had instituted a program of walking patients even while they were on ventilators. Traditionally, patients on ventilators are left in bed with their hands restrained to prevent them from reaching out and pulling out the breathing tube; we also keep them heavily sedated to prevent those kinds of accidental occurrences. In Giffords's case we would stop her sedation in the morning and our rehab people, respiratory therapists, nurses, and doctors would start the rehabilitation processes, even though she was still on the ventilator. Within a few days she was able to sit up in bed and dangle her legs over the side, and after a week she was able to briefly stand up by her bedside with the aid of the ICU nurses. Later the ICU nurses started taking her in a wheelchair up to the helicopter landing pad on the hospital roof so she could get a panoramic view of the city she loved. Whenever she was moved, she was equipped with a specially designed helmet to protect her brain.

Eventually I removed her ventilator tube, inserted a tracheostomy tube, and a tube directly into her stomach, which made her more comfortable and allowed us to remove her feeding tube from her nose, but she still was unable to speak. I invited two Navy ophthalmologists I knew from San Diego to come in to discuss the surgical repair of her damaged right eye socket; eventually it was reconstructed with titanium mesh, screws, and pieces of shattered bone. I upgraded her official condition from critical to serious.

In the meantime, Mark Kelly and I were considering plans for her eventual transfer to a rehabilitation facility. I was pushing hard for The Institute for Rehabilitation and Research (TIRR) Memorial Hermann–Texas Medical Center in Houston.

There were several reasons for that. One was that TIRR is a world-class institution, probably the best rehab facility in the country. Another was that the head of trauma at Memorial Hermann–TMC was my longtime friend and colleague Dr. John Holcomb, a retired Army colonel and former commander of the US Army Institute of Surgical Research—and he was the best in the business. He had been the premier Army surgeon when he was on active duty, and he had set up a program in Houston to train military medical personnel in a civilian trauma center, just as I had in Los Angeles; John probably did more for military trauma training than anyone in my era. As a former military trauma surgeon and researcher, John had had extensive experience in the treatment of traumatic brain injuries—far more than his civilian counterparts, in fact. I knew he would take good care of her until she started rehab.

But there was another reason why I wanted Gabby to go to Houston—and that was because of Mark Kelly.

After the shooting, Mark had advised NASA to pick a backup commander for the upcoming Space Shuttle *Endeavour* mission scheduled for April. Given the circumstances, he wasn't sure he would be able to fly the mission, and he didn't want to jeopardize its success.

That was understandable. I had gotten to know Mark in the days after the shooting, and I admired his fierce determination to take care of his wife and ensure she got the best possible care. I also admired his calm strength in dealing with an incredibly difficult situation. He was and is a good man.

But as a former Navy captain myself, I also believed that for him to give up a mission he had spent the past two years training for would be devastating, not only for himself but perhaps also for Gabby. It wasn't Mark's first space mission—he had flown three already—and there was no doubt that NASA would appoint a competent replacement if necessary. He kept saying, "I've been there before."

But I was convinced that as a military man, Mark would inevitably feel that dropping out of the mission would be letting everyone down, including himself and his wife. I also knew Navy jet pilots. I knew that he and Gabby would regret it if he didn't go. I was also concerned that it might cause Gabby to experience feelings of guilt that could hinder her recovery. I have often seen patients go through feelings of guilt about their injuries, even if they'd had nothing to do with them. They start feeling like a burden to their loved ones, that they've disrupted everybody's lives, which only adds to their depression. That was the last thing I wanted Gabby to experience.

But Mark couldn't picture going on the mission while his wife needed him. It wasn't even an option. I tried to convince him that by the time the mission took place she would be fine, and it would not only be good for him to go but it would also be good for the country. But even though he wanted to go, he wasn't budging. He had no idea how well she was going to be doing that spring.

So I knew that if she went to a rehabilitation facility other than in Houston, he would not be going on his mission. Which is why as subtly as I could I steered him toward TIRR, which would allow him to remain close to her while still training for the mission. The decision was ultimately his, but I was glad when he decided that Gabby would go to Houston for rehab, and he was going back to NASA.

A word here about rehabilitation programs. I've said over and over in this book that in my trauma center, everybody gets treated the same. And that's true. But sadly, after patients leave the trauma center, they often face inequities in their extended care. Many of my patients are young people or poor people without health insurance, and they simply don't get the rehab care that those who have insurance or can afford it receive.

For example, about a month after the Giffords shooting I had a woman with a nearly identical injury come into our trauma center. She was about the same age as Gabby and had been shot in the brain. She was a mother and had a loving and supportive family; it seemed like half a dozen members of her family were at her bedside in the ICU the entire time she was there. She got the same care in my trauma center as the congresswoman did, with nearly identical results. The difference was she didn't have health coverage, and she wasn't even a US citizen. So ultimately I had to discharge her to her family and not to an expensive rehab center, which could have added immeasurably to her recovery. Later the family took her back to Mexico, and to this day I wonder how she did.

Of course, I'm glad that Gabby was able to receive the best possible rehabilitation. I just wish everybody could. I wish that we had a system that could have given that other woman the same treatment, a system based on medical necessity and compassion, not on money. I'm sure Gabby and Mark feel the same.

Anyway, on January 21, thirteen days after the shooting, the congresswoman was taken by ambulance from University Medical Center to Tucson's Davis-Monthan Air Force Base. Hundreds of people lined the ambulance route, cheering and waving American flags. At the air base she was put aboard a Challenger jet, accompanied by Mark, several nurses, and a Capitol Hill police officer. Randy Friese also went with her—and in a way so did I. The wireless cuff monitor that I had earlier developed with NASA and Athena GTX was hooked up to her and would transmit her heart rate, blood pressure, and pulse. Giffords was among the first civilian patients to benefit from the use of this new device, which after testing by the military had been approved by the FDA and had gone on the civilian market shortly before the shootings. Again, for a scientist and researcher, it's always satisfying to see your work help a patient in the field.

With the congresswoman's departure, the public spotlight inevitably shifted. The reporters and TV crews all packed up and went elsewhere; the deluge of thousands and thousands of cards and letters that had poured in began to trail off. I didn't regret it. I thought that the UMC Trauma Center team had performed magnificently under the public scrutiny, and that the public had gained some understanding and appreciation of what trauma surgery in general is all about.

But what I think most people didn't understand was that except for the number of victims and the press of the crowds and the TV cameras, for those of us in the trauma community— surgeons, nurses, EMTs—the Tucson mass shooting really was not all that unusual. In a perfect world it wouldn't be so. But the reality in this country is that there are always going to be people who have been shot, stabbed, bludgeoned, crushed in a car accident, or otherwise gravely injured and desperately in need of help.

And whether the public spotlight is on or off, every minute of every day we are ready for them—ready for the next life-or-death catastrophe that comes rushing in through the swinging doors. It's what we train for, what we plan for, what we do.

EPILOGUE

Congresswoman Gabby Giffords continued her slow but steady process of recovery. In February she spoke her first word, which the media reported was *toast*, as in, she wanted toast with her breakfast of yogurt and oatmeal. Later Mark told me her actual first word was *what*, spoken a few days earlier, but it didn't really matter. From small beginnings come great things. Soon thereafter she was speaking phrases—including, like most patients long confined to a hospital, the phrase "Want to get out of here."

Her rehab wasn't easy. While in Houston she had to undergo another surgery, in which surgeons replaced the missing parts of her skull with a ceramic material. Like most brain-injury patients, she also suffered intense frustration at the slow pace of recovery. Nor did her rehab cease when she left TIRR after five months. It would continue for years.

And yet compared with what most of the world expected on that morning in January 2011, her recovery was miraculous. In May she traveled to Florida to watch Mark and his crew launch their successful last *Endeavour* Space Shuttle mission. In August she returned to the floor of the House of Representatives to cast a vote for a debt-ceiling bill and was greeted with an emotional standing ovation. Later, in 2012, she led the Pledge of Allegiance at the Democratic National Convention in Charlotte, North Carolina.

The other wounded victims also began their lives again. Ron Barber, Giffords's district office manager, successfully ran to replace her in Congress after Giffords announced in 2012 that she was resigning to concentrate on her recovery. Pam Simon, the congresswoman's community outreach director, is busier than ever and stays in contact with me.

The shooter, meanwhile, underwent extensive psychological testing before ultimately pleading guilty and being sentenced to life without parole. His was another life wasted.

As for me, the spotlight from the Tucson mass shooting didn't really change my life, but it did make it busier in some ways.

On January 25, 2011, I was honored to sit in the presidential box at the State of the Union address as a guest of Michelle Obama. The two dozen other guests included military service members; several high school science prodigies; Daniel Hernandez Jr., the young congressional intern who had rushed to the congresswoman's side after the shooting; and John and Roxanna Green, the parents of Christina-Taylor Green. Later that year Emily and I were invited to a White House state dinner for then–South Korean president Lee Myung-bak.

However, those honors were eclipsed still later when I went back to Uniontown, Pennsylvania, to be inducted into the Life Achievement Hall of Fame at Laurel Highlands High School, my alma mater. State of the Union addresses and gala White House dinners are nice, but for a formerly shy, geeky Korean kid to be honored by his old high school was something special. I had never been sorry that I had left Uniontown for a life of study and travel and adventure, but I was pleased that my old hometown thought I had done well.

Education and travel and adventure are things that I always try to promote to young people. They can be the difference between a life you look back on with regret and one you can look back on with satisfaction and a sense of accomplishment.

In fact, those were the themes I stressed when I was invited to give the commencement address to the University of Arizona class of 2012. I briefly told the five thousand graduates and their proud parents and family members in the packed arena about my first plane ride when I was six, about growing up in Uganda, about my father's relentless commitment to education and the admiration I felt for my parents. I told them about my own desire to get out and see the world, about the satisfaction of serving as a Navy trauma surgeon, about the Marine we lost on Pearl Harbor Day in Ramadi. I told them that they could find some good in every day, even in such little things as having a fresh, clean Porta-John on a cold December morning in Iraq. I told them that no matter what anybody said, no matter how gloomy things might appear, every day was a good day.

"Today is a good day," I told the graduates. "I know that when you look or listen, you will hear about the wars around the world, the hungers, the pains, the war on drugs, global warming, border issues, the inequities, failing economies, the loss of jobs, budget cuts to education and health care. There are forty to fifty million Americans with no health insurance, the jobs are tough to get, and so on and so on. Seemingly the world is imploding today or tomorrow. According to the news, it's only going to get worse.

"But I say, 'Look around you. What do you see?' In an airplane, when the gauges all tell you that you are falling out of the sky, the first thing you are taught to do is look out the cockpit and see if the instruments are correct. Let me tell you what I see when I look out the cockpit today. Life is good and it is getting better. I see educated people graduating. I see people who will make the world better and not worse. Education is responsible for our progress in civilization. Look at the unbelievable accomplishments made in the last three decades alone . . . We can do many things today that we could not even imagine when I graduated from college. Yes, today is a good day. When everyone is convinced that our world is spiraling downward toward impending implosion, look outside the cockpit and see if those gauges are correct. I say they are not. It looks great outside. It is sunny, and there are five thousand smarter people graduating today, and over ten thousand proud family and friends who can attest that today is a good day."

My involvement in the Tucson shootings also thrust me into a role as a public advocate—for commonsense gun-control measures, for the restructuring and improved funding of trauma treatment in this country, and for trauma surgery in general.

Not long after the shooting I wrote a newspaper editorial, one that was picked up nationally, about the need for improved background checks on gun purchasers. To me that sounded like a simple thing, one that wouldn't violate anyone's Second Amendment rights while making it more difficult for troubled individuals like the Tucson shooter to obtain firearms and ammunition.

I got a lot of negative reaction to it from people who thought I was advocating taking their guns away, or that I didn't know anything about guns. That wasn't true. As a military man, I've been around guns all my adult life. And I'm still a gun owner. But a lot of people feel the same way I do. Not only was a proposal in Congress to tighten up the background checks supported by a host of prominent politicians and individuals, including Mark Kelly and Gabby Giffords, but polls showed it was supported by an overwhelming majority of the American people, including a majority of gun owners. And yet somehow, as of this writing, it still hasn't been accomplished.

But if we as a nation aren't going to take even the most simple of actions to regulate firearms, we should at least be aware of what that level of freedom is costing us.

Sure, people pay attention to the cost of gun violence when there is a mass shooting like the one in Tucson and later in the movie theater in Colorado and the horrific killing of school-children at Sandy Hook Elementary School. For a few days or weeks after such mass-casualty events, we as a nation are riveted on the terrible human cost of gun violence.

But what most people don't realize is that, as terrible as they are, such mass shootings account for only a tiny fraction of the gun deaths and wounds in this country. The vast majority of people shot in this country are shot in ones and twos and threes. And although in the aggregate their numbers are astonishing—again, thirty thousand firearm deaths in America every year—most people don't even hear about them. There might be a line or two on the local TV news—"A man was shot and killed today on the city's south side"—but that's about it. And to be frank, whatever side of town the man was shot in is usually the side of that town that most people don't really care about. Believe me, if the thousands of gun homicides that take place in America were happening on supposedly safe suburban streets, as they did that day in Tucson, even the politicians would have to do something about it.

But they don't. The vast majority of Americans have never seen a gunshot wound, and they never will. It's frustrating for me, because as a trauma surgeon I see the cost of gun violence almost every single day—not just in the bodies of the shooting victims, but in the anguished faces of their families and friends.

The good news for people who get shot or violently injured in America—if there's any good news in being shot or violently injured—is that unlike thirty or forty years ago, we now have a system of Level I trauma centers that are staffed and equipped to save their lives. Again, a seriously injured person has a 25 percent better chance of survival if he makes it to a Level I trauma center than if he's taken to an ordinary ER or a hospital with a lower level of trauma care available.

Unfortunately, there are still some serious problems with our trauma care system.

One big problem is that there aren't enough trauma surgeons to go around. That's partly because of the lengthy and demanding residency and training requirements for surgery in general, and trauma surgery in particular, and partly because of the long hours being a trauma surgeon demands. We can't do anything about the first; trauma surgery is always going to take a long time to learn. After twenty years I'm still learning things I didn't know before. But maybe we can do something about the long hours on the job.

As I mentioned earlier, regulations now limit residents to eighty hours per week, and I think we need to do the same for other members of the medical profession, trauma surgeons included. It would mean we would make less money, and patients would have to get used to the idea that the surgeon who operated on them might not be available to them during their recovery. But the problem is that the older you get and the more experience you have as a trauma surgeon, the less able you are to handle the physical stress of working the crazy hours that we do. If the working hours allowed for a reasonable home and social life, maybe more medical students would get into the field—and we need as many good ones as we can get.

Another big problem with our trauma system is funding. Again, we spend only a tenth as much of our national health costs on trauma as we spend on other illnesses, despite the fact that trauma is the number-one cause of death among children and the number-one cause of death among all Americans under the age of forty-eight. Same thing goes for trauma research, the finding of new ways to save traumatic injury patients—including, for example, the suspended-animation process I described earlier. Trauma research saves lives—someday maybe including your own.

We could fix the problems in trauma funding by making trauma center care a social service and not a fee-for-service—in other words, with public funding for the operation of trauma centers. As it now stands, trauma centers are private entities that depend on patients who can pay—that is, the ones who have health insurance—to take up the slack for the many trauma patients who can't pay. In the end we all get hit with higher insurance rates. Meanwhile, trauma centers have to spend an inordinate amount of time hassling with insurance companies and trying to raise money through private fund-raisers. The constant search for money negatively affects the quality of medical care.

Instead, as a nation or as states within the nation, we should establish a steady public revenue stream to finance trauma care and research. Some states already do that, at least partially. In the state of Maryland, for example, ten dollars out everyone's annual car license fee is earmarked to support the state's trauma centers. Since cars are involved in so many trauma injuries, maybe we could put a tax of a couple of cents per gallon on gas to support trauma centers. By the same reasoning, maybe we could put a penny tax for trauma research on each of the seven to ten billion rounds of ammunition sold in this country every year. It wouldn't cost an individual very much, but it could go a long way in preventing and treating trauma deaths.

The problem with getting the taxpayers to support public

funding for trauma centers is that most taxpayers don't think that they or their loved ones will ever need one. A lot of us worry ourselves sick about getting cancer or heart disease, but how many people wake up thinking they might get shot or be injured in a car crash that day? Despite the statistics, most Americans don't see trauma as a major national health issue.

But trauma is a major health issue—and not just here in America. As part of my public advocacy work in the wake of the Tucson shootings, I've also tried to spread the word about the importance of trauma treatment systems in other countries, including the country of my birth, South Korea. Like most other highly developed countries in Asia and Europe, South Korea doesn't have anything near the violent assault rate that we have in this country, especially violence involving guns. South Korea strictly regulates private gun ownership, so in an average year it will have about ten gun-related incidents leading to death or injury—not ten thousand, not ten hundred, but ten.

But South Korea and other advanced countries still have trauma—from accidents, suicides, and car crashes. So I've been working with the South Korean government to develop a trauma care system. I hope to be able to do the same in other countries.

In fact, I've become sort of a wandering preacher for the cause, traveling around the country and the world and speaking out about the individual and public health benefits of advanced trauma care systems. For me that's an easy sell, because as I hope I've made clear in this book, I not only believe in what I do, I also love what I do. Sometimes I can hardly believe I get paid to do it.

Yes, the hours are tough, and I have to travel a lot for professional reasons, and I have to deal with some pretty horrific situations. It can be exhausting and frustrating and heartbreaking, and it's hard to have a normal family life. But the ironic thing is that the reasons I could hate the job are the same reasons I love the job. Every day is different, I get to see things that most people never see, I get to travel around and deliver a message I fervently believe in. It's challenging, exciting, exhilarating.

And most important, I get to help people. As I said earlier, I strongly believe that no one in the world needs somebody more than someone who has been shot or stabbed or crushed in a car accident needs a trauma surgeon. It's an honor for me to be there for them.

So I guess I can sum it up by saying that despite the many twists and turns in my professional life, I was born to be a trauma surgeon.

And as I look back on it, I wouldn't have wanted to be anything else.

ACKNOWLEDGMENTS

First and foremost I would like to thank my wife, Emily, and my children, Michael and Anna, for learning to eat dinner between nine and ten P.M. Although I have missed many Christmases and birthdays, it was always for the right reasons.

My thanks also to my brother, who suggested this book; to Crystal Kasnoff, who believes in me and encouraged me to do this project that she managed; and to my cowriter, Gordon Dillow, who worked diligently to smooth out some of the rough edges. My thanks also to Colin Harrison at Scribner for believing in this book, and to Katrina Diaz for helping to put it together.

Many remarkable people appear in the pages of this book, and to them I want to express my gratitude and admiration. They include former congresswoman Gabrielle Giffords and her husband, former astronaut and Navy Captain Mark Kelly, and other survivors of the Tucson mass shooting, who set a new standard for courage, resilience, and strength; the doctors, nurses, and staff at University Medical Center in Tucson, who excelled that day as they excel every day; the first responders of Tucson and Pima

County, Arizona, and first responders everywhere; and the men and women of the US military, past and present, who allowed me the honor of serving with them as a Navy officer.

Behind the scenes are my fellow surgery partners at UMC, my work family, who are the best and are solely responsible for making me look good at times, and Laura Ballesteros, my "work wife," who is responsible for everything, as I have no value without her. My thanks and admiration also to Kari, for showing me how to behave in front of important people; to the nurses at UMC, especially the ones in the trauma bays, the OR, and 2DW; my boss, Dr. Rainer Gruessner, who never ceases to amaze me with his endless support and belief in me; Dr. Tom Wachtel, who dedicated his life to trauma and helped rescue the trauma program in Tucson; and the people of Tucson, who have taken me in as their own and have been more generous than words can describe.

Thanks also to Chuck S., my most long-standing friend ever; Stephen Dawkins, for inspiring my interest in medicine; Mike M., my bestest travel buddy who shared all my adventures in med school; Steve Bell, we shared more adventures than we can remember and with whom I'll never stop laughing; Drs. Ken Waxman and Gail Tominaga, role models who got me interested in trauma; Drs. Maier, Jurkovich, and Gentiello, who helped me so much in my career; Captain Stu Markey for teaching me about the world; Dr. Norman Rich for the endless opportunities that he has given me; Dr. Hasan Alam, who helped me with my experiments and my success; Dr. Geoff Ling, who owes me a son; Dr. Demetriades, my LA boss and friend; George V, who is the best surgeon and worst tennis player; Kenji, the most loyal friend; Carlos, Matt, and Ali, my LA connection buddies; Dr. Ken Mattox, who has been the most influential and pivotal surgeon; Marty Schrieber and John Holcomb for their friendship

ACKNOWLEDGMENTS

and service to the Army; all the fellows whom I had the privilege of influencing against their will; my fellow academic trauma surgeons, who had to endure this book so others would have an idea of what the heck we do for a living; and to all those with whom I had the privilege of serving in both war and peace.

PHOTO CREDITS

INDEX

ABOUT THE AUTHORS

Dr. Peter Rhee is Chief of Trauma, Critical Care, Emergency Surgery, and Burns at the University of Arizona Medical Center and a tenured professor of surgery. He spent twenty-four years on active duty in the US Navy, including combat tours as a forward-deployed surgeon in Afghanistan and Iraq, before retiring in 2007 with the rank of captain. An internationally renowned researcher and lecturer, Dr. Rhee has pioneered developments in the fields of traumatic hemorrhagic shock and resuscitation, hemostatic products, advanced portable electronic medical devices, and the use of suspended animation in the treatment of trauma victims. He and his wife, Emily, live in Tucson with their children, Michael and Anna.

Gordon Dillow has been a reporter, columnist, and war correspondent for more than thirty years. He has written for a number of newspapers, including the *Orange County Register*, the *Los Angeles Times*, and the *Los Angeles Herald Examiner* and is the coauthor of *Where the Money Is* and *Uppity*. He lives in Scottsdale, Arizona.